A Guide to
Neonatal Care

Acknowledgements

Figures 3.1 and 14.3 are copyright © 2009 Royal College of Paediatrics and Child Health.

Figure 5.1 was created by BruceBlaus and can be found here: https://commons.wikimedia.org/wiki/File:Hand_Hygiene.png. This file is licensed under the Creative Commons Attribution-Share Alike 4.0 International licence.

We are grateful to Daniel Roberts for his kind permission to reproduce Figures 8.1, 8.8, 11.7, 11.12, 11.16, 12.1 and 12.2, plus the images within Table 9.2.

Figures 8.2 and 11.4 have been reproduced with the kind permission of Resuscitation Council UK.

Figure 9.8 is sourced from Lindsay Mgbor/Department for International Development and can be found here: www.flickr.com/photos/dfid/7497732174. This is reproduced under CC BY 2.0 DEED.

Figure 14.2 was created by Yehudamalul and can be found here: https://en.wikipedia.org/wiki/Small_for_gestational_age#/media/File:Weight_vs_gestational_Age.jpg. This file is licensed under CC BY-SA 3.0.

To order our books please go to our website www.criticalpublishing.com or contact our distributor Ingram Publisher Services, telephone 01752 202301 or email IPSUK.orders@ingramcontent.com. Details of bulk order discounts can be found at www.criticalpublishing.com/delivery-information.

Our titles are also available in electronic format: for individual use via our website and for libraries and other institutions from all the major ebook platforms.

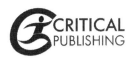
CRITICAL
PUBLISHING

A Guide to
Neonatal
Care
Handbook
for health
professionals

Julia Petty, Sheila Roberts and Lisa Whiting

First published in 2024 by Critical Publishing Ltd

British Library Cataloguing in Publication Data
A CIP record for this book is available from the British Library

ISBN: 978-1-915080-50-9

This book is also available in the following e-book formats:
EPUB ISBN: 978-1-915080-51-6
Adobe e-book ISBN: 978-1-915080-52-3

Text design by Greensplash
Cover design by Out of House Limited
Project management by Newgen Publishing UK
Printed and bound in the UK by 4edge Limited

Critical Publishing
3 Connaught Road
St Albans
AL3 5RX

www.criticalpublishing.com

Contents

Meet the editors

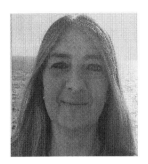

Julia Petty began her children's nursing career at Great Ormond Street Hospital, London, in 1988. After a period in paediatric and neonatal clinical practice and education, she moved into higher education and worked as a senior lecturer at City University, London, for 12 years, co-leading the neonatal nursing post-registration education portfolio. She commenced her current role at the University of Hertfordshire as senior lecturer in child nursing in 2013 and has been Associate Professor (learning and teaching) since 2020. One of the modules she leads focuses specifically on caring for the neonate and family. Julia's key interests are neonatal nursing care and health, the parent experience, outcome of early care and, most recently, the development of digital storytelling resources in children's nursing care and education.

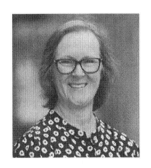

Sheila Roberts qualified as a general and children's nurse in 1983 and started her career at Birmingham Children's Hospital before moving into general paediatrics in a range of hospital settings. She moved into education in 2006 and has since been responsible for teaching and assessing pre-registration BSc (Hons) children's nursing students at the University of Hertfordshire across a range of modules, from practice to health promotion, anatomy and physiology to research. As admissions lead for children's nursing, she has given children a voice in selecting suitable candidates to join the children's nursing programme, by inviting them to interview candidates. She has been involved in research evaluating the role and value of the NHS England Youth Forum, which gives young people a voice within healthcare services, and was also involved in a study with families who have children with complex needs, exploring the parents' resilience both before and after an intervention was implemented.

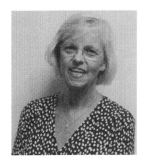

Lisa Whiting is Associate Dean for Research, Associate Professor [Research] and, at the time of editing this book, Professional Lead for children's nursing at the University of Hertfordshire. She qualified as a general and children's nurse in 1983 and then primarily worked for several years within a paediatric critical care setting. In her current post Lisa is involved in the teaching and assessing of undergraduate and postgraduate students across a range of academic levels. She completed her own doctorate in 2012 and since then has led several research projects that have spanned a range of child and neonatal health issues and that have had a strong focus on the involvement of, and the voice of, children, young people and their families. Other research has centred on the enhancement of learning for nurses working within areas of child health and children's nursing. Lisa supervises doctoral students whose work focuses on aspects of nursing and midwifery well-being, child health and patient care.

Meet the contributors

Karen Afford is a trained health visitor and now works as a Senior Lecturer for the MSc/PGDip/BSc Specialist Community Public Health/Nursing programmes (Health Visiting/School Nursing Community/Children's Nursing/District Nursing/General Practice Nursing) at the University of Hertfordshire.

Melanie Carpenter is trained as an Advanced Neonatal Nurse Practitioner (ANNP) and is also an Independent and Supplementary Prescriber. Currently, she works as the Assistant Professor of Midwifery at Coventry University, Course Director for the Midwifery BSc and Lead Midwife for Education. She is also responsible for leading the neonatal qualified in speciality (QIS) and newborn and infant physical examination courses.

Jo Day is a lecturer in Children and Young People's Nursing at the College of Nursing and Midwifery, Birmingham City University. She is responsible for the education of both undergraduate and postgraduate nursing students. Her particular interests are early attachment and bonding, breastfeeding and perinatal mental health. As a registered specialist community public health nurse and educator, she aims to deliver family-centred care allowing parents and carers to feel supported throughout their parenting journey.

Emmie Hopkinson is a newly qualified children's nurse who has a particular interest in paediatric mental health and emergency care. She successfully completed her BSc Children's Nursing degree at Kingston University in 2023 as well as the highly regarded Council of Deans for Health Student Leadership programme.

Nadia Lawes is a senior lecturer in the School of Health and Social Wellbeing, College of Health, Science and Society, at the University of the West of England. She currently works in children's nursing education. Her clinical background has been focused primarily around critical and intensive care nursing, both in the UK and abroad. She has experience within paediatric anaesthetics, recovery, neurosurgery, paediatric and neonatal intensive care.

Laura Maguire is Pathway lead – Neonatal critical care, Senior Lecturer, College of Nursing and Midwifery, Birmingham City University. She qualified as a registered children's nurse in 2009 and then worked on a neonatal intensive care unit for nine years. Laura now leads the post-registration neonatal critical care pathway.

Kathleen Mangahis is Senior Lecturer in Children's Nursing and pathway lead for the Neonatal Nursing/QIS modules at Kingston University. She has over 20 years of neonatal care experience and is specialised in neonatal surgery as a particular area of interest.

Louise McLaughlin is a senior lecturer who joined the Children's Nursing team at the University of Hertfordshire in 2022. She has a special interest in children's palliative care having worked in children's hospices for 14 years.

Katy Moss started working in neonatal care after qualifying as an adult nurse in 2010. She qualified as a Neonatal/QIS nurse in 2014 by completing a BSc (Hons) Neonatal Care degree and now works as a Sister/Team leader at the Neonatal Unit, Lister Hospital, East and North Hertfordshire NHS Trust. Her particular areas of interest are patient/family-centred care and improving the neonatal journey for our small patients and their families.

Karen Roberts-Edema is a senior lecturer in Children's Nursing at the University of Hertfordshire with over 10 years' experience in children's community nursing. She has a specialist interest in children with complex care needs in the community and is a Queen's Nurse, a highly acclaimed recognition for expertise in this area.

Michelle Scott is an Advanced Neonatal Nurse Practitioner at the Neonatal Unit, University Hospitals Coventry and Warwickshire, with 20 years of neonatal care experience. She is interested in education, neonatal haemodynamic and 'Point of Care' Ultrasound Scanning (POCUS).

Laura Watson is a Professional Nurse Advocate and a senior lecturer in children's nursing with a specific responsibility for neonatal-focused education at the University of the West of England. Prior to this, she worked across all levels of neonatal care including tertiary surgical, cardiac and neurological care. Laura has a strong interest in supporting breastfeeding and partnership working with families.

Preface

Julia Petty

BOOK OVERVIEW

This textbook is a practical guide to the care of neonates and families within clinical and community settings from birth up to the first year of life. The purpose of this book is to serve as a guide for clinical care, containing information to support practice for health professionals working with neonates and infants. It is not the intention of this book to give lengthy explanations or protocols, nor is it intended to replace approved policies. Rather, it aims to offer a 'snapshot' reference guide to support knowledge in clinical care with reference to relevant literature and national guidelines where applicable. In this way, the book aims to be universally applicable to anyone caring for neonates and/or infants in the clinical and/or home setting.

TERMINOLOGY AND INCLUSIVITY

As a general rule, the book uses the word 'neonate' for the period up to 28 days of life (post term) and 'infant' for up to one year, although the terms will be used interchangeably throughout the text. Use of the word 'baby' will pertain to the newborn period at birth. The word 'parent' is used throughout to include caregivers, carers and anyone with parental responsibility for infants from any ethnic, cultural and/or religious background. The book also uses the words 'mother', 'father', 'woman' and 'man'; while it is accepted these are gendered terms, their use is inclusive of any parent who identifies as female or male, including trans women and trans men whose gender may be different to the sex assigned at birth. Therefore, terminology used in the book is consistent with the guidance from the National Institute for Health and Care Excellence (2023) that uses the terms 'woman' or 'mother' throughout, taken to include people who do not identify as women but are pregnant or have given birth.

In relation to 'family', the UK Office for National Statistics (2023) refers to a married, civil partnered or cohabiting couple with or without children, or a lone parent with at least one child. However, the book recognises this is a traditional, 'nuclear' family definition and that we must also recognise 'non-traditional' families, eg blended families, separated, divorced, and same-sex couples, families with adopted, foster, or stepchildren.

Regarding ethnic diversity, reports have highlighted that women and neonates from a racially minoritised background (EMBRACE-UK, 2023), or from poorer backgrounds, are disproportionately affected by health inequality, which has a direct impact on health and outcomes in neonatal care (National Health Service Race and Health Observatory (NHSRHO), 2023). A NHSRHO review highlighted that it is vitally important to consider the specific assessment practice for neonates/infants from ethnically diverse backgrounds who have non-Caucasian skin tones, identifying specific factors that must be considered when assessing Black, Asian and/or minority ethnic neonates. Where applicable, reference will be made to these specific observances within the book, to ensure an inclusive approach to assessment and care of all neonates, whatever their background, race, ethnicity and skin tone.

BOOK STRUCTURE

The book is divided into four main sections. The introduction discusses the importance of clinical, practice-based learning in neonatal care, placing this in the context of the holistic care of the infant and family. A discussion on the application of clinical guidance for neonatal practice then follows, within an evidence-based approach. Part 1 covers care of the healthy neonate and infant, including anatomy and physiology, basic care principles, normal development, assessment, screening and important healthcare practices within the context of the family. Part 2 covers clinical neonatal care, including the neonatal unit and hospital setting, while Part 3 focuses on care of the infant and family at discharge and beyond at home in the community setting.

It is acknowledged that local thinking and guidance will invariably affect certain practices, which may influence the applicability of certain parts of this guide at the local unit level. Therefore, where necessary, reference should be made to any relevant local protocols or formal practice guidelines in your own clinical area and workplace. By drawing on the general guidance offered by this book alongside your own local variations, we hope this book will be a contextual and relevant resource to support practice and learning. This can provide an additional opportunity for learning and further discussion. Health professionals should learn from each other across different disciplines or neonatal settings, acknowledging that practice variations may exist. The main message is that whatever specific guidelines are followed, we all aim for the same outcome: that of optimising care and minimising risk to our vulnerable neonates and their families.

HOW TO USE THIS BOOK AND THE WEB COMPANION

The book is intended to support essential learning in neonatal care. Chapters are formatted in a consistent way, including a main title, sub-sections, key learning objectives, critical thinking points, various guides for learning (labelled as figures or tables), a range of 'alert' boxes with symbols and a reference list with relevant supporting literature. The learning guidance is in one of four formats: summary tables, checklists, flow charts or information boxes with illustrations where appropriate. The 'stop and think' alert boxes highlight important practice points of clinical significance or areas of caution. 'Standard precautions' alerts are included where appropriate, in line with prevention of cross-infection. Cross-referencing between chapters is provided indicated by a 'signpost' icon to direct the reader to related topics. A 'local variations' alert box at the end of each chapter reminds the reader to check their own workplace specific guidance with additional space to note their personalised local practices.

Cross-referencing is also made throughout the text to a web-based book companion hosted on the publisher website. On this web platform, each chapter has its own glossary to explain relevant definitions and abbreviations along with other resources and supplementary information as appropriate.

The web companion can be accessed at www.criticalpublishing.com/skills.

Key to figures, tables and symbols

Figures and tables	
	Checklist
	Flow chart, photograph or diagram
	Summary table
	Information box

Alert boxes and symbols	
	Stop and think – highlights important points, cautions or any areas of controversy.
	Standard precautions – where applicable, this symbol highlights important infection control reminders.
	Signpost – links with related chapters and topic areas are highlighted by this symbol throughout the book.
	Web-based information – refer to the book's web companion material for supplementary content. The web companion can be accessed at www.criticalpublishing.com/skills; ebook readers using a suitable device can click or tap to access this directly.
	Local variations – this symbol is used with space below it to record any local variations and practice points specific to your own unit or place of work.

REFERENCES

EMBRACE-UK (2023) MBRRACE-UK Perinatal Confidential Enquiry: A Comparison of the Care of Asian, Black and White Women Who Have Experienced a Stillbirth or Neonatal Death. [online] Available at: www.npeu. ox.ac.uk/mbrrace-uk/reports#mbrrace-uk-perinatal-confidential-enquiry-a-comparison-of-the-care-of-asian-black-and-white-women-who-have-experienced-a-stillbirth-or-neonatal-death (accessed 28 January 2024).

National Health Service Race and Health Observatory (NHSRHO, 2023) Review of Neonatal Assessment and Practice in Black, Asian and Minority Ethnic Newborns: Exploring the Apgar Score, the Detection of Cyanosis and Jaundice. [online] Available at: www.nhsrho.org/research/review-of-neonatal-assessment-and-practice-in-black-asian-and-minority-ethnic-newborns-exploring-the-apgar-score-the-detection-of-cyanosis-and-jaundice/ (accessed 28 January 2024).

National Institute for Health and Care Excellence (NICE) (2023) NICE Style Guide: Talking about People. [online] Available at: www.nice.org.uk/corporate/ecd1/chapter/talking-about-people (accessed 28 January 2024).

Introduction

Julia Petty

NEONATAL CARE IN CONTEXT

Within the field of neonatology, a multi-disciplinary team comprising a range of healthcare professionals may provide care for sick neonates and their families; the team may include nurses, health visitors, doctors, paramedics, midwives, speech therapists, physiotherapists, social workers, dieticians, pharmacists, psychologists and religious figures. This is congruent with the importance of interprofessional learning, an essential component of current healthcare education. Interprofessional learning occurs when two or more professions learn with, from and about each other to improve collaboration and the quality of care. It focuses on the needs of individuals, families and communities in order to improve their quality of care, health outcomes and well-being, keeping best practice central throughout all teaching and learning. The care required by neonates and their families in the hospital and community setting can be complex, meaning there is much to learn for those working in this field. The past few decades have seen significant changes in the role of the neonatal healthcare team, as well as considerable technological developments, changes in the education of specialty training and ongoing clinical research (National Health Service (NHS), 2019). Along with advances in neonatal care that contribute to the improvements seen in neonatal outcomes, learning needs are diverse and knowledge acquisition relating to the nuances of neonatal care is essential (Petty et al, 2019, 2022).

 See the web companion for supplementary information relating to the context of neonatal care.

The focus of this book is on providing a guide for clinical care of the neonate within the hospital and community setting. However, when caring for neonates in any setting, it is important to have knowledge about the healthy neonate to serve as a baseline for assessment and care when clinical intervention is needed. Moreover, fundamental care principles must not be forgotten in relation to treating neonates as individuals within a family care context.

DIVERSITY AND INCLUSIVITY

The neonate, like any service user of the healthcare system, should be respected as an individual. This not only includes their physical needs but also their psycho-emotional, social, spiritual and cultural needs. Care must be *culturally sensitive* (Kaihlanen et al, 2019), recognising, for example, diversity of ethnic background, gender preference, sexual orientation and religious observances of the whole family. The delivery of interventions must consider the neonate's and family's individuality; this includes background, social-economic status, gestation, age, underlying condition and family context, in order to tailor care most appropriately.

Importantly, we, as editors, emphasise how essential it is to ensure diverse and inclusive guidance. Families must have equitable care and we must value, celebrate and embrace equity, diversity and inclusion (EDI) in line with the Equality Act 2010 and the protected characteristics detailed within it. These are (listed alphabetically and not in relation to to any priority): age, disability (to include physical and learning disabilities as well as, although arguably not a disability, neurodiversity), gender reassignment, married or in a civil partnership, pregnancy or being on maternity leave, race including colour, nationality, ethnic or national origin, religion or belief, sex and sexual orientation.

THE NEONATE WITHIN THE FAMILY INTEGRATED CARE CONTEXT

It should be emphasised that any individual, specific care practice must be delivered within a family integrated approach. This should always be at the forefront of neonatal practice as it has shown to be effective at reducing maternal parental stress and anxiety (Cheng et al, 2021). Children at any age, including neonates, are best cared for by their parents or certainly in a partnership approach between healthcare professional and parents/carers. This approach should include planning of care, negotiation of who will give that care and how primary carers for that neonate can participate as much as possible (Brødsgaard et al, 2019). The topic of family integrated care in practice is covered later within this book.

THE IMPORTANCE OF CLINICAL GUIDANCE TO SUPPORT NEONATAL CARE

Teaching in the clinical setting, and particularly bedside teaching is viewed by patients, students and educators as an invaluable teaching method (Burgess et al, 2020). A learning guide can be defined as a tool a learner uses to work through concepts or processes while demonstrating their think-ing, planning and/or decision making on the way to understanding and con-solidating knowledge.

INCORPORATING EVIDENCE TO SUPPORT NEONATAL CARE

The application of recent and valid evidence in the neonatal field is an essential part of delivering best practice to the neonate and family. It is also integral to effective learning so that knowledge is delivered and assimilated by the learner within the context of what the evidence has shown. Neonatal care has a scientific base upon which to base care, and great strides have been made in translating research into practice in this specialty. Examples are the introduction of new ventilation techniques including non-invasive modes, the advent of surfactant and antenatal steroids in the light of evi-dence linking these to improved outcomes, and the implementation of both developmental care and inclusive, family-integrated care principles into neonatal care delivery that recognises diverse groups and people. Learning tools therefore should also have a grounding within this evidence-based perspective.

REFERENCES

Brødsgaard, A, Pedersen, J T, Larsen, P and Weis, J (2019) Parents' and Nurses' Experiences of Partnership in Neonatal Intensive Care Units: A Qualitative Review and Meta-synthesis. *Journal of Clinical Nursing*, 28 (17–18): 3117–39.

Burgess, A, van Diggele, C, Roberts, C and Mellis, C (2020) Key Tips for Teaching in the Clinical Setting. *BMC Medical Education*, 20: 463.

Cheng, C, Franck, L S, Ye, X Y, Hutchinson, S A, Lee, S K and O'Brien, K (2021) Evaluating the Effect of Family Integrated Care on Maternal Stress and Anxiety in Neonatal Intensive Care Units. *Journal of Reproductive and Infant Psychology*, 39(2): 166–79.

Kaihlanen, A M, Hietapakka, L and Heponiemi, T (2019) Increasing Cultural Awareness: Qualitative Study of Nurses' Perceptions about Cultural Competence Training. *BMC Nursing*, 18: 38.

National Health Service (NHS) (2019) *Implementing the Recommendations of the Neonatal Critical Care Transformation Review*. [online] Available at: www.england.nhs.uk/publication/implementing-the-recommen dations-of-the-neonatal-critical-care-transformation-review (accessed 5 December 2023).

Petty, J, Jarvis, J and Thomas, R (2019) Understanding Parents' Emotional Experiences for Neonatal Education: A Narrative, Interpretive Approach. *Journal of Clinical Nursing*, 28(9–10): 1911–24.

Petty, J, Whiting, L, Fowler, C, Green, J and Mosenthal, A (2022) Exploring the Knowledge of Community-Based Nurses in Supporting Parents of Preterm Babies at Home: A Survey-Based Study. *Nursing Open*, 9(3): 1883–94.

Part 1

Caring for the healthy neonate and family

Section editors: Sheila Roberts and Lisa Whiting

1 Understanding neonatal anatomy and physiology

Emmie Hopkinson and Julia Petty

INTRODUCTION

An understanding of neonatal physiology shapes an individual's approach to the care they deliver to the patient (Griffiths et al, 2021). Therefore, it is important to understand neonatal-specific anatomy and physiology with the aim of accurately differentiating between a 'normal' assessment and any potential abnormalities (Petty, 2011a). The neonatal period is one of dramatic physiological changes. Transition of a newborn baby to extra-uterine life is a critical time to adapt to life outside the uterus (Doherty et al, 2023). Respiratory and cardiovascular systems change immediately at birth (Table 1.1, Figure 1.1), while other systems evolve and change throughout neonatal life and infancy until early childhood, continuing until the transition from intrauterine to adult physiology is complete. Thus, physiology is different in young children, especially in neonates and infants, from that of older children and adults (Saikia and Mahanta, 2019) (Table 1.2).

Chapter learning objectives

By the end of this chapter you will:

✓ have gained an overview and understanding of the key differences between typical neonatal anatomy and physiology as compared to older children and adults;

✓ have gained an insight into the normal transition to extra-uterine life at birth.

Critical thinking points

• Consider what vital observations and physiological signs you may visually encounter in neonates/infants.

• What are the key points in neonatal anatomy and physiology that would affect the nursing care you deliver?

See Chapter 4 for a systems approach to *assessment* specifically and Chapter 7 for the related *altered* physiology of the neonate/infant.

 See the web companion for supplementary information on transition at birth.

TRANSITION AT BIRTH

At birth, the newborn baby undergoes a transition to an extra-uterine environment and must adapt from being a foetus to a neonate who lives independently from placental transfusion of oxygen and nutrition. Successful transition depends on the availability of adequate oxygen, energy in the form of glucose and adequate thermal control. This occurs in most neonates when born healthy (Aylott, 2006, cited in Turnbull and Petty, 2013).

 Table 1.1 Physiological changes at birth

- The loss of the low-pressure placenta and its ability to facilitate gas exchange, circulation and waste management for the foetus creates a need for physiological adaptation (Doherty et al, 2023).

- There is increased systemic vascular resistance following separation from the placenta.

- Closure of right-to-left shunts occurs, namely:

  - foramen ovale (closes when left atrial pressure is greater than right atrial pressure);

  - ductus arteriosus (left-to-right flow within minutes of breathing, then closure over days).

- Rapid lowering of pulmonary vascular resistance occurs with onset of breathing.

- Clearance of fluid from airways takes place via active sodium absorption and changes in airway pressure due to ventilation.

- An increased metabolic rate leads to higher glucose needs and glucose homeostasis adaptation occurs (see web companion).

- Increased catecholamine levels support blood pressure.

- Fluid distribution changes (see web companion).

(Adapted from Morton and Brodsky, 2016; Doherty et al, 2023)

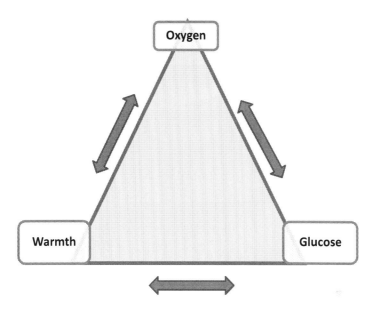

 Figure 1.1 The Metabolic Triangle: physiological requirements at birth

---

🖐 *Stop and think*

The neonate requires early provision of all three of these areas for successful adaptation to extra-uterine life, from delivery room and thereafter.

OVERVIEW OF NEONATAL ANATOMY AND PHYSIOLOGY

A systems approach is useful to consider how the anatomy and physiology of neonates and infants differs from that of older children and adults.

⊞ Table 1.2 Neonatal-specific anatomy and physiology (compared to older child/adult)

System	Features
Respiratory	• Neonates have smaller, shorter and less efficient lungs. As the neonate grows, larger lungs will be more effective and will increase in capacity to compensate for conditions such as hypoxia.
	• Increased basal metabolic rate = higher oxygen consumption.
	• Neonates will become tachypnoeic in response to hypoxia.
	• Higher (normal) respiratory rate between 40 and 60 breaths per minute (bpm) (compared to child average 15–40 bpm).
	• Epiglottis is floppy and situated at a higher position.
	• The narrowest part of the airway is the subglottic region at the cricoid.
	• The airway is funnel shaped (becomes cylindrical after eight years old).
	• The diaphragm is the main respiratory muscle. Intercostal muscles are developing and therefore are less effective as accessory muscles.
	• Shorter necks, smaller mouths, narrow nares and larger tongues = less airway protection.
	• Thorax is softer with a greater proportion of cartilage, meaning lower elastic recoil during breathing.
Cardiovascular and haematological	• Neonates are less efficient in reserves to effectively manage compromise and illness.
	• Myocardium and autonomic control of the heart is immature.
	• Less contractile heart with lower myocardial reserve.
	• Cardiac output is dependent on rate rather than stroke volume.

System	Features
	• There is higher pulmonary vascular resistance in the first few weeks of life.
	• Heart rate variability ranges vastly between resting and active values (approx. 70 to 190 beats per minute).
	• Total blood volume is low (85 ml/kg).
	• There are higher haematocrit and haemoglobin levels in the newborn period.
	• Red blood cells have a shorter life span of approximately 60–70 days. This can increase the risk of physiological jaundice.
	• There is no vitamin K production until the neonate is fully fed.
	• Liver immaturity can lead to extended clotting times.
Immune	• Immunoglobulins start to produce in-utero mid-trimester, with transfer across the placenta starting in the last trimester.
	• Neonates will not receive the full transfer of immunoglobulins across the placenta during the last trimester if born prematurity, which will cause them to be further immunocompromised.
	• Neonates have less effective phagocytic action and impaired opsonic activity with relatively reduced complement levels.
Digestive	• The digestive tract is structurally complete but functionally immature due to reduced levels of certain digestive enzymes in the first 9–12 months.
	• Gastric acid production is lowered with extended gastric emptying.
	• The cardiac sphincter of the stomach is frequently weak, predisposing the neonate to gastro-oesophageal reflux.
	• The first feed triggers postnatal changes in the function of the gastro-intestinal tract so that hormones are stimulated and the gut matures. Until feeding is established, the neonate can rely on sudden cessation of glucose via the placenta and alternative substrates such as ketones for energy and metabolism. Following metabolic adaptation and the first feed, glucose comes from an exogenous source and levels normalise.

Table 1.2 (cont.)

System	Features
Hepatic	• Immature liver and hepatic enzyme systems result in a slower rate of the metabolism of endogenous and exogenous substances such as breakdown of heme to bilirubin.
	• There is a reduced formation of clotting factors.
	• Physiological jaundice due to liver enzyme immaturity is a common risk.
	• A delay in establishing feeding can lead to a slow digestive transit time, which can lead to increased reabsorption of bilirubin back into the hepatic pathway and the circulation.
Fluid balance/ renal and urinary-genital	• Kidney development is complete by week 36 of pregnancy except for the nephrons which continue to mature for longer.
	• There is a relatively low glomerular filtration rate (GFR) until approximately one year of age. This means an inferior response to excessive fluid load with the kidneys unable to tolerate large volumes, as well as a lower ability to concentrate urine and excrete excess acids, solutes or drugs and toxic waste.
	• At birth, a contraction of the extracellular fluid volume occurs in the immediate postnatal period to adapt to extra-uterine life.
	• 75 per cent of the birth weight is total body water with a higher extracellular to intracellular fluid ratio.
	• Approximately 10 per cent of the total body weight is lost postnatally.
	• External genitals should be fully developed, and sex differentiation should be clearly visible at birth.
	• Male – the testes should have descended into the scrotum and are palpable with the scrotal skin showing deep rugae.
	• Female – the labia majora should cover the labia minora and clitoris.
Thermoregulatory	• Neonates have an immature thermoregulatory system and a greater disposition to heat loss.
	• The hypothalamus, which is the central control centre for thermoregulation, is immature and can lead to an inability to generate heat physiologically.

System	Features
	• They have a high surface area to volume ratio with relatively large heads, which is a site of potentially high heat loss through exposure to cooler environmental air temperature or convective air currents, radiation towards cooler surfaces and through direct contact with cold surfaces by conduction.
	• Newborn babies have wet skin which can easily lead to significant and rapid heat loss through evaporation.
Metabolism	• Neonates have a higher basal metabolic rate (BMR), necessitating a much higher glucose and oxygen need.
	• High energy demand is required for a high rate of growth.
	• Neonates have more limited glycogen stores and may also lack nutritional reserves (fat, iron and vitamins) which are developed within the third trimester of pregnancy.
	• Glycogen stores are more easily exhausted in response to compromise.
Neurological	• The brain comprises a higher percentage of total body weight with a much higher glucose requirement for growth.
	• The central and peripheral nervous systems are not fully developed at birth unlike the automatic nervous system.
	• Myelination is yet to be fully developed within the central nervous system. Development of more refined co-ordination, motor and development skills, along with higher cognitive functions, continue to mature over the childhood period.
	• Typically, neonates demonstrate reflexive behaviours in the early weeks. The presence of reflexes such as Moro, ventral suspension, sucking, rooting, grasp (palmar), plantar and tonic reflexes indicate normality in the central nervous system.
	• Over time, the higher centres within the cortex will take precedence over the reflexive primitive behaviours. The neonate learns to engage in purposeful movements and actions while the reflexes diminish.
	• Anterior and posterior fontanelles on the surface of the head indicate soft skull sutures that have not fused, allowing for early brain growth.

$\longrightarrow$

Table 1.2 (cont.)

System	Features
Sensory	• Senses are fully intact and continue to mature over the first few months.
	• From birth, a 'typical' neonate will be able to see, hear, taste, smell, respond to touch and feel pain.
	• Neonates have the ability to fix on and follow an object or face from birth at a distance of no greater than 20 centimetres. Full visual acuity is developed at approximately six months.
	• The 'red reflex' should be elicited on a formal examination, which shows reflection from the retina through the pupils that should constrict to light rapidly and equally on both sides.
	• Neonates' heads turn to sound, and they will startle.
	• They are responsive to positive touch, kinaesthetic stimulation (eg rocking) and skin-to-skin contact, all of which can soothe and console.
	• Neonates are responsive to pain stimuli by exhibiting key pain cues – crying, bulging of the brow, grimace of the face and eyes, agitation, tensing and increased heart rate.
	• They have the ability to differentiate different tastes (sweet/sour) and can smell breast milk and their parent's skin.
Behavioural	• There are different behavioural states: deep sleep, light sleep, fussiness, awake/alert and crying/active.
	• Neonates have the ability to state regulate or self-console through shutting down their central nervous system enough to block out excessive stimuli (also known as 'habituating' to external stimuli).
	• Physiologically, state regulation involves tightly flexed limbs with little movement and the neonate sleeping with hand-to-mouth action.
	• Stimulation should take place when the neonate is in a quiet, alert state.
Musculoskeletal	• Physiological flexion occurs at approximately 34 weeks' gestation where the foetus has developed good muscular tone.
	• During this period of gestation, they are positioned with arms and legs tucked up in a flexed, mid-line position, the characteristic posture of a healthy term neonate following delivery.

System	Features
	• Hip joints should show adequate movement through both abduction and adduction as they have fully developed with the pelvic bone.
Integumentary	• Skin should be fully developed, intact, clear and smooth.
	• Term neonates have a well-developed stratum corneum complete with keratin formation.
	• Vernix caseosa is commonly seen, consisting of fatty secretions from foetal sebaceous glands and dead epidermis cells forming protection.
	• Skin should feel centrally warm with adequate perfusion (capillary refill time ideally less than 2–3 seconds in conjunction with other signs). Mucous membranes should be pink (eg lips, tongue, gums) rather than observing skin, to allow for a diverse range of skin tones across various ethnicities.
	• Skin can be sensitive to external agents which can commonly cause rashes, such as milia and erythema toxicum. However, these do not usually cause a problem or require treatment.
	• The 'acid mantle' of newborn skin serves as natural protection against infection, which ideally should not be eliminated using early or regular bathing with alkaline products.
	• Early or regular bathing with alkaline products may also lead to delayed separation of the umbilical cord due to delay in normal skin flora colonisation.
	• The umbilical cord stump and surrounding skin should look clean and dry and separate within 5–15 days of life.

(Adapted from Petty, 2011a, b, c)

 Stop and think

Neonates are not just small children! They have a unique anatomy and physiology that develops and matures further as they age into children.

 See the web companion for a glossary specific to this chapter.

📍 *Check local variations and guidance alert*

The space below can be used to record any notes or local variations and practice points specific to your own unit.

REFERENCES

Doherty, T M, Hu, A and Salik, I (2023) Physiology, Neonatal. StatPearls Publishing. [online] Available at: https://pubmed.ncbi.nlm.nih.gov/30969662 (accessed 31 October 2023).

Griffiths, N, Laing, S, Spence, K, Foureur, M and Sinclair, L (2021) The Effects of Nurse-Delivered Caregiving in the Neonatal Setting: An Integrative Review. *The Journal of Neonatal Nursing*, 27(5): 317–26.

Morton, S U and Brodsky, D (2016) Fetal Physiology and the Transition to Extrauterine Life. *Clinics in Perinatology*, 43(3): 395–407.

Petty, J (2011a) Fact Sheet: Neonatal Biology – An Overview Part 1. *The Journal of Neonatal Nursing*, 17: 8–10.

Petty, J (2011b) Fact Sheet: Neonatal Biology – An Overview Part 2. *The Journal of Neonatal Nursing*, 17: 89–91.

Petty, J (2011c) Fact Sheet: Neonatal Biology – An Overview Part 3. *The Journal of Neonatal Nursing*, 17: 128–31.

Saikia, D and Mahanta, B (2019) Cardiovascular and Respiratory Physiology in Children. *Indian Journal of Anaesthesia*, 63(9): 690–7.

Turnbull, V and Petty, J (2013) Evidence-based Thermal Care of Low Birthweight Neonates. Part One. *Nursing Children and Young People*, 25(2): 18–22.

2 Fundamental neonatal care principles

Nadia Lawes and Laura Watson

INTRODUCTION

Newborn infants are reliant on others to meet their needs in terms of maintaining cleanliness and comfort and minimising the risk of infection. Healthcare professionals have an important role to support the infant's parents and primary caregivers in developing their confidence and competence to carry out personal care in response to their infant's cues. This chapter provides an overview of eye, mouth, umbilical, nappy (Tables 2.1 to 2.5) and skin care alongside bathing guidance. It is also important for healthcare professionals to be able to identify 'normal' childhood conditions and to distinguish these from more serious illnesses such as jaundice, gastro-oesophageal reflux and skin rashes (Tables 2.6 to 2.8).

Chapter learning objectives

By the end of this chapter you will:

✓ have gained an overview of the personal care needs of the healthy term neonate;

✓ have been introduced to some common neonatal conditions.

Critical thinking points

- Consider the importance of providing appropriate and safe personal care in relation to infection prevention.

- Identify the links between personal care giving and carer involvement/bonding.

 See Chapter 8 for further detail on the topics in this chapter in relation to neonatal unit care: namely, skin care, hygiene needs and jaundice.

See the web companion for supplementary information on fundamental care of the healthy neonate/infant.

 Check local guidance

Personal care in relation to any of the areas covered in this chapter should follow specific local guidance.

PARENT PARTICIPATION

While undertaking personal care for their infant, parents should be encouraged to develop their confidence through participation and moving towards leading care. Information should be available to ensure parents understand any proposed intervention. Formal consent is not usually requested or required but staff should be attentive for signs of assent, such as body language; this includes consideration of the infant's cues and signs of readiness.

EYE CARE

Routine eye care is not generally required, but may be indicated:

○ to prevent, or treat, infection;

○ to remove visible debris or encrustation;

○ to prevent and relieve pain or discomfort;

○ to prevent dryness and damage to the eyes; for example, post-surgery, when eye coverings are used, during continuous positive airway pressure (CPAP) or when receiving muscle relaxants.

 Table 2.1 Eye care guideline

When eye care is indicated, a clean technique and effective handwashing should be utilised to minimise the risk of introducing infection.

• Gather equipment: personal protective equipment (PPE) (gloves, apron), rubbish bag, sterile gauze swabs, ampoules of sterile saline and sterile container for cleaning liquid.

Table 2.1 (cont.)

- Explain the procedure to parents/carers and obtain consent.
- Ensure that lighting is appropriate but not directly pointed at the infant's eyes and position them appropriately.
- Wash hands and put on clean gloves.
- Assess condition of the infant's eyes, monitoring for signs of infection.
- Pour sterile saline into container, if applicable.
- Clean the least affected eye first.
- Using a clean, moistened swab/wipe to clean from inner canthus (nasal corner) to outer canthus, and clean lower and upper lids from nose to side.
- Repeat with a new swab each time until all discharge has been removed.
- Wipe excess moisture from the surrounding skin.
- Ensure the infant is calm and comfortable, considering their position in line with local developmental care guidance.
- Document care and condition of the infant's eyes, reporting any concerns regarding potential infection to the medical team and parents.

 Standard precautions alert

Dispose of waste according to local policy and wash your hands, ensuring that excess saline is not disposed of in handwashing sinks (applies to all hygiene care).

 Stop and think

'Sticky' eyes, yellowish discharge which may dry on the eyelid, can be caused by blocked tear ducts and are not necessarily an indication of infection (Bowen and Taylor, 2021). Signs of infection may include erythema, localised oedema (not related to birth trauma), changes to the lining of the lower lid and purulent discharge.

 Standard precautions alert

If infection is suspected, a swab may be indicated, medical review requested and topical treatment commenced.

MOUTH CARE

Provision of regular mouth care ensures ongoing oral health, maintaining comfort, providing positive oral stimulation for infants and supporting sensory development of taste and smell (Bruce et al, 2023). If expressed breast milk/colostrum is used, the infant will have further benefits associated with maternal milk. Bruce et al (2023) highlight that both the frequency and equipment utilised for oral care are frequently debated in the literature.

The aims of mouth care are to:

○ maintain a clean and healthy oral cavity;

○ keep mucosa moist;

○ maintain lip health;

○ promote comfort of the infant.

Local guidelines will support the frequency of mouth care for babies admitted to the neonatal unit and further adjustments to the outline below. Some units may advocate for routine use of liquid paraffin during mouth care (Thames Valley & Wessex Network, 2019).

Mouth care should be individualised for the infant, responding to their behavioural cues, sleep cycle and ability to tolerate handling. When undertaking mouth care, it is important to assess the condition and appearance of the infant's lips, mucous membranes, tongue and saliva. Ensure that their lips and mucous membrane are pink, smooth and moist, recording any signs of cracking, redness, ulceration or presence of oral candida.

Table 2.2 Mouth care guidelines

- Gather appropriate equipment: PPE (non-sterile gloves and apron), sterile gauze, cotton applicators, sterile water, colostrum/expressed breast milk and waste bag/container.
- Wash your hands and apply PPE.
- If indicated, perform oral suction under direct vision before performing mouth care.
- Dampen gauze with sterile water/maternal expressed breast milk, removing excess, and clean the infant's lips – seeking to remove debris.
- Dispose of gauze and repeat if required.
- Apply colostrum to gauze/applicator and roll slowly across the lips.
- In relation to applicator/gauze, this can also be rolled along gum line and over the tongue.
- Ensure the infant is calm and comfortable, considering their position according to local developmental care guidance.
- Document the care and condition of the infant's mouth, reporting any concerns regarding potential infection to the medical team and parents.

Stop and think

Foam applicators are not recommended for mouth care because they are too large to enable gentle and responsive care for babies. Further, an National Patient Safety Agency alert was issued in 2012 following an adult death where the sponge detached from the handle during use.

CARE OF THE UMBILICUS

The umbilical cord, which is clamped and cut at birth to leave the umbilical stump, initially appears white, plump and moist. It will dry, then gradually shrivel and change to a dull brown, before turning black and then detaching completely – usually from 5–15 days after birth.

⊞ Table 2.3 Principles of umbilical care

- The umbilical stump provides a favourable medium for bacteria. A number of evidence-based strategies have been proposed to minimise infection, including cleaning with antiseptic solutions.
- Recent analysis of the available evidence, however, has found that antiseptic agents may delay drying of the cord and subsequent detachment.
- Parents should be encouraged to wash their hands before handling their infant's umbilical stump, and to keep it clean and dry. Washing should preferably be undertaken with water only, although mild soap can be used if the stump becomes contaminated with urine or faeces.
- After bathing, the stump should be patted dry with a clean towel and allowed to completely dry before putting on the nappy.
- Advise parents to fold down the front of the nappy to avoid physical irritation and to allow the umbilical stump to remain dry and free from contamination.
- The cord base remains vulnerable to infection even after the cord detaches and until it is completely healed, which takes several weeks. During this time care should continue to be taken to maintain cleanliness and observe for signs of infection.
- Also observe the umbilical area for signs of granuloma or hernia.

 Standard precautions alert

Ensuring the umbilical stump stays clean and dry is essential to prevent infection. Regular observations are needed of the site to check for redness or discharge that may indicate infection.

Umbilical infections can occur, and potential routes of infection include colonisation via the birth canal and from direct contamination during or soon after delivery. Most infections are caused *by Staphylococcus aureus*, although Group A and B Streptococci and *Escherichia coli* are other common pathogens. Serious complications may occur because of umbilical infection because it provides a direct access to the blood-stream (Stewart and Benitz, 2016).

 Table 2.4 Signs of omphalitis

- Skin surrounding the stump appears red and/or hot to touch.
- Presence of discharge.
- Fever.
- Distress when stump is handled.
- Infant appears unwell and lethargic, with poor feeding.

 Stop and think

The process which the umbilical cord undergoes is one of dry gangrene, and as such odour is not unexpected. Malodour **alone** does not indicate omphalitis (Wheeler, 2016).

Some babies are at particular risk of developing omphalitis. Risk factors include low birth weight; unplanned home delivery; prolonged rupture of membranes and chorioamnionitis during the pregnancy (Stewart and Benitz, 2016). Be particularly vigilant in babies with one or more risk factors and maintain a low threshold for investigation/referral.

CARE OF THE SKIN AND BATHING

When caring for the infant, attention should be paid to preserving the unique 'acid mantle' which babies are born with. At birth, and for the first four days, the skin has an acid pH, and this is important in protecting the newborn from infection. In addition, the skin is covered in specific proteins, which provide further protection. It is therefore important to minimise disruption of these natural defences. It is generally advised that bathing is not undertaken immediately after birth and that daily baths are not required, with two to three times per week considered sufficient. Washing with plain water is preferable, or with pH-neutral products if needed. Bath water temperature should be

37 degrees Celsius at a depth no more than 2–3 cm. Hair should be washed first, keeping the infant wrapped (Figure 2.1) and then the body is exposed to place them in the bath. Tolerance and signs of stress should be observed for while always holding the infant (Figure 2.2). The infant is lifted safely from the bath by placing an arm under their body, clasping the furthest upper arm firmly and holding both ankles with the other hand (Figure 2.3).

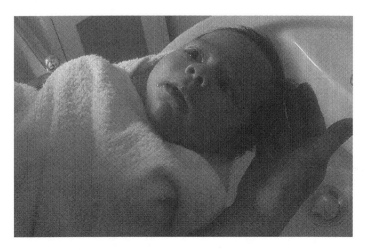

↗ Figure 2.1 Hair washing before baby bath

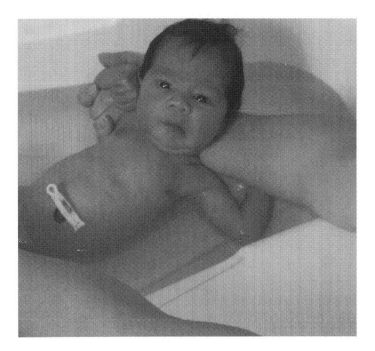

↗ Figure 2.2 Bathing baby

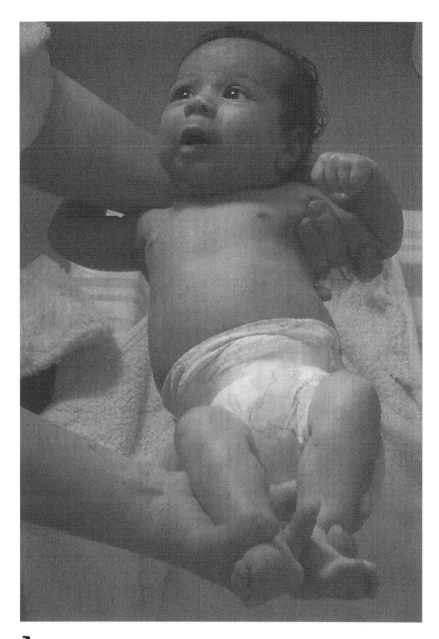

 Figure 2.3 Lifting baby from the bath

✋ *Stop and think*

Although it is important to be mindful about the appropriateness of bathing, remember that it is often a positive experience and an important opportunity for parent interaction, promoting bonding.

NAPPY CARE

Neonates may pass urine between 5 and 20 times a day and open their bowels after every feed (Bruce et al, 2023). While modern nappies are absorbent, prolonged periods in a moist environment leads to the skin becoming increasingly fragile. Further, the reaction between urine and faeces creates ammonia, which increases skin pH and can lead to a breakdown of the skin barrier (Bowen and Taylor, 2021) as well as susceptibility to damage from friction on the skin. This results in red and inflamed skin, nappy rash, which increases the neonate's discomfort and increases the risk of acquired infection.

Table 2.5 Nappy care guidelines

- Explain procedure to parents/carers and gain consent.
- Gather appropriate equipment: PPE (non-sterile gloves and apron), cotton wool/ non-sterile gauze, small bowl, waste bag, clean nappy and water (as per local guidance).
- Wash your hands and apply PPE.
- Put water into a bowl.
- Ensure the neonate is on a safe, flat surface.
- Undress the neonate to gain access to the nappy.
- Remove the dirty nappy and place it into a waste bag.
- Using a moistened cotton ball/gauze, clean genitalia from front to back to reduce the risk of infection. Ensure the skin is not pulled, potentially causing trauma.
- Dispose of used cotton ball/gauze in a nappy bag and repeat on the other side of genitalia until clean.
- Gently clean between the fold of the groin and thigh, and then the buttocks.
- Gently pat dry the area with dry gauze/cotton ball.
- Place a clean nappy under the neonate and secure, ensuring a boy's penis points downwards. Consider what is appropriate elevation of the legs depending on the neonate's gestation.
- Ensure the umbilical stump is positioned outside the nappy.
- Redress the neonate.
- Nappies may be weighed to provide information regarding fluid balance.
- Ensure the neonate is calm and comfortable, considering their position according to local developmental care guidance.
- Document nappy care and condition of the skin, reporting any concerns regarding potential infection to the medical team and parents.
- Dispose of soiled nappy according to local policy and wash hands thoroughly after dealing with body fluids.

The use of products within the water, or baby wipes, is not required and is generally avoided (Bruce et al, 2023); this helps to reduce disruption to skin pH as well as irritation and sensitivity. Where nappy rash is present, topical treatment may be necessary either to treat excoriation or as a barrier against further trauma. Treatments will vary according to local guidance and should be discussed with the medical team.

COMMON NEONATAL CONDITIONS

It is important to have an awareness of some of the common conditions which can affect the neonate. You should be able to inform parents and carers, observe and monitor improvement or deterioration, and be vigilant for signs of more significant issues.

⊞ Table 2.6 Care of the neonate with jaundice

- Jaundice or hyperbilirubinaemia refers to high levels of bilirubin in the bloodstream. Bilirubin is a yellow-coloured bile pigment that can accumulate and become visible within the skin, sclera of the eyes and/or mucous membranes (eg gums). Importantly, given poor visual detection of jaundice in Black and darker skin toned neonates (National Health Service (NHS) Race and Health Observatory, 2023), it is vital to not rely solely on skin assessment.

  ☛ See Chapter 8 for further detail on assessment including that relating to ethnic diversity and skin tone.

- Jaundice is common in newborns, with approximately 60 per cent of term babies experiencing it within the first week of life (National Institute for Health and Care Excellence (NICE), 2010).

- Bilirubin is produced by the breakdown of red blood cells. Initially, bilirubin exists in an *unconjugated* form, which cannot be excreted. In order to be removed from the body, unconjugated bilirubin must first be bound to albumin and transported to the liver, where it can be metabolised to form *conjugated* bilirubin. Conjugated bilirubin can then be carried in bile through the gut and excreted via the stool.

- Newborn babies can experience jaundice because they have an increased number of red blood cells, which have a shorter than usual lifespan. Their liver function is also immature.

- For most neonates with jaundice, this is classed as *physiological* (associated with the normal adaptations of the body after birth) and does not require treatment. However, any neonate with jaundice should have their bilirubin levels assessed using a transcutaneous bilirubinometer, or via a blood test, to determine if treatment is required.

- Initial treatment is through phototherapy, which uses blue light to directly convert the unconjugated bilirubin into an excretable form without the need for metabolism in the liver.

- Jaundice can also be caused by other conditions, such as sepsis, metabolic disorders or blood group incompatibility between the mother and neonate.

- If levels of unconjugated bilirubin were to exceed albumin-binding capacity, 'free bilirubin' can penetrate the blood–brain barrier and cause direct damage to neurological tissue, although this is rare.

Stop and think

Breastfed neonates are more likely to develop physiological jaundice than those who are fed with formula (Huang et al, 2023). The reasons for this are not well understood, although it is thought to be related to overall intake, gut activity, increased reabsorption of bilirubin via the gut or specific factors within the breast milk itself. However, jaundice should not be a reason to stop breastfeeding and mothers should be suitably informed and offered lactation support.

⊞ **Table 2.7 Care of the neonate with gastro-oesophageal reflux**

- The term reflux is used to describe the involuntary regurgitation of the stomach contents into the oesophagus.

- Gastro-oesophageal reflux is common, affecting around 40 per cent of infants (NICE, 2015). It is characterised by frequent episodes of effortless regurgitation of feeds, not associated with burping.

- Infants are at increased risk of reflux because the sphincter between the oesophagus and the stomach is immature. Premature neonates and those with complex neurodevelopmental disorders are also more commonly affected.

- Gastro-oesophageal reflux is often benign and self-limiting, and can be managed through parental support, offering smaller, more frequent feeds, or thickening feeds.

- Many cases resolve by one year of age as the sphincter matures and the diet is no longer primarily fluid-based.

- If gastro-oesophageal reflux becomes problematic (exhibited by poor weight gain and/or distress) and requires medical treatment, it is classed as gastro-oesophageal reflux disease (GORD). These two terms are often used interchangeably but are in fact distinct from one another.

- GORD is commonly diagnosed clinically, although in some cases investigations such as a pH study may be undertaken.

 Stop and think

Be aware of red flags in neonates who are vomiting as this can be an indication of a more serious condition. These red flags include:

- projectile vomiting;

- bile-stained or blood-stained vomit;

- signs of dehydration or lethargy;

- faltering growth.

⊞ Table 2.8 Rashes in the neonatal period

Rashes in the neonatal period are common and it can be difficult to distinguish normal rashes from those caused by more serious conditions. It is important to understand the terms used to describe the characteristics of rashes.

- *Macules* are flat lesions.

- *Papules* are raised lesions up to 1 cm in size.

- *Nodules* are raised lesions between 1 cm and 2 cm in size.

- *Vesicles* are raised lesions filled with clear fluid which are less than 1 cm in size.

- *Pustules* are raised lesions filled with pus (Lissauer and Claydon, 2018).

Common causes of rash

- **Milia** – also known as 'milk spots'. Small keratin-filled cysts which appear as small white papules on the face and scalp or on the roof of the mouth, and which resolve spontaneously within a few weeks.

- **Miliaria rubra** – caused by obstruction of sweat glands and appearing as small red papules and vesicles – commonly referred to as 'heat rash'.

- **Erythema toxicum neonatorum (ETN)** – usually appears within the first three to four days, sometimes referred to as 'baby acne'. The aetiology of ETN is unclear but it is thought to be caused by the accumulation of inflammatory cells around infected hair follicles. ETN appears as macules and papules which develop into pustules on an erythematous (reddened) base.

- **Seborrheic dermatitis** – red and scaly in appearance. It is caused by a hormone-related increase in sebaceous gland activity. Seborrheic dermatitis is usually noted initially on the scalp (often called cradle cap), sometimes also spreading onto the face and behind the ears.

- **Atopic dermatitis** – felt to be related to an exaggerated immune response and alterations within the protective functions of the epidermis. It is often associated with later diagnoses of asthma and allergy. Atopic dermatitis is characterised by redness, oedema and the presence of vesicles which burst, causing oozing and subsequent crusting. It is usually found on the face and scalp, as well as the extensor surfaces of the arms and legs. Atopic dermatitis may require treatment in the form of emollients.

(Reynolds et al, 2022)

Stop and think

It is important to be able to recognise signs and symptoms of any neonatal condition in all skin tones and ethnicities, recognising that they may be more difficult to identify in darker skin tones (NHS Race and Health Observatory, 2023), for example identification of erythema, cyanosis and jaundice.

Many textbooks describe and illustrate only examples of assessment on white skin. *Mind the Gap* by Mukwende et al (2020) is an invaluable resource dedicated to describing and demonstrating clinical signs in black and brown skin tones.

In addition, refer to the NICE guidance on postnatal care for further recommendations on a range of care considerations in the newborn baby (NICE, 2021).

 ## Standard precautions alert

Wash your hands thoroughly before and after providing personal care to prevent cross-infection, especially during eye and umbilical cord care.

 See the web companion for a glossary specific to this chapter.

 ## Check local variations and guidance alert

The space below can be used to record any notes or local variations and practice points specific to your own unit.

REFERENCES

Bowen, R and Taylor, W (2021) *Skills for Midwifery Practice*. Oxford: Elsevier.

Bruce, E, Williss, J and Gibson, F (2023) *The Great Ormond Street Hospital Manual of Children and Young People's Nursing Practices*. 2nd ed. Chichester: Wiley-Blackwell.

Huang, H, Huang, J, Huang, W, Huang, N and Duan, M (2023) Breast Milk Jaundice Affects Breastfeeding: From the Perspective of Intestinal Flora and SCFAs-GPR41/43. *Frontiers in Nutrition*, 10: 1121213.

Lissauer, T and Claydon, W (2018) *Illustrated Textbook of Paediatrics*. 5th ed. Oxford: Elsevier.

Mukwende, M, Tamony, P and Turner, M (2020) *Mind the Gap: A Handbook of Clinical Signs in Black and Brown Skin*. London: St George's University of London.

National Health Service (NHS) Race and Health Observatory (2023) Review of Neonatal Assessment and Practice in Black, Asian and Minority Ethnic Newborns: Exploring the Apgar Score, the Detection of Cyanosis and Jaundice. [online] Available at: www.nhsrho.org/research/review-of-neonatal-assessment-and-practice-in-black-asian-and-minority-ethnic-newborns-exploring-the-apgar-score-the-detection-of-cyanosis-and-jaundice (accessed 28 January 2024).

National Institute for Health and Care Excellence (NICE) (2010, updated 2023) Neonatal Jaundice. [online] Available at: www.nice.org.uk/guidance/cg98 (accessed 1 November 2023).

National Institute for Health and Care Excellence (NICE) (2015) Gastro-oesophageal Reflux Disease in Children and Young People: Diagnosis and Management. NICE Guideline [NG1]. [online] Available at: www.nice.org.uk/guidance/ng1 (accessed 1 November 2023).

National Institute for Health and Care Excellence (NICE) (2021) Postnatal Care. NICE Guideline [NG194]. [online] Available at: www.nice.org.uk/guidance/ng194/chapter/Recommendations#postnatal-care-of-the-baby (accessed 1 November 2023).

Reynolds, S, Punia, H, Harrison, L B and Rodriguez-Garcia, C (2022) A Guide to Neonatal Rashes. *Paediatrics and Child Health*, 32(12): 463–70.

Stewart, D and Benitz, W (2016) Umbilical Cord Care in the Newborn Infant. *Pediatrics*, 138(3): e20162149du.

Thames Valley & Wessex Network (2019) *Guideline Framework for Mouth Care on the Neonatal Unit*. [online] Available at: www.piernetwork.org/uploads/4/7/8/1/47810883/mouth_care_guideline_-_final.pdf (accessed 1 November 2023).

Wheeler, B (2016) Health Promotion of the Newborn and Family. In Hockenberry, M, Wilson, D and Rodgers, C (eds) *Wong's Essentials of Pediatric Nursing*. 10th ed (pp 190–228). St Louis: Elsevier.

3 Developmental aspects of the healthy neonate

Laura Watson and Nadia Lawes

INTRODUCTION

Even within the first 28 days of life, important advances are already taking place in an infant's development and their progression towards increasing independence. Although there are some individual variances in attainment of milestones, it is important to have a working understanding of expectations for age, because the failure to meet milestones may indicate an underlying issue. This chapter covers growth (including weight patterns and the use of growth charts to plot weight) as well as developmental influences and milestones including reflexes (Figures 3.1 and 3.2; Tables 3.1 to 3.4), as they apply to the healthy term infant in the first year of life.

Chapter learning objectives

By the end of this chapter you will:

✓ have considered the importance of accurate growth monitoring;

✓ have been introduced to newborn reflexes and developmental expectations for the healthy term infant in the first year of life.

Critical thinking points

- Consider factors that can influence neonatal development, including those which are individual to the infant and those related to their environment.

- Explore the responsibility that healthcare professionals have to advise parents on the growth and development of their infant and how to signpost them to appropriate support.

For growth and development relating to the premature infant in the neonatal unit and after discharge home, please refer to Chapter 14.

GROWTH

Birth weight is influenced by factors such as maternal health during pregnancy, maternal size and ethnicity, with smoking having an adverse effect (British Nutritional Foundation et al, 2013).

In the first few days of life, babies will lose weight due to fluid loss and the use of fat stores while feeding is being established (Toro-Ramos et al, 2015). Guidelines from the National Institute for Health and Care Excellence (NICE, 2017) regarding faltering growth identify that the loss of up to 10 per cent of birth weight within the first three days is common. NICE suggests, however, that healthy term infants who continue to lose weight after day 4 or those who have not returned to birth weight by three weeks of age should be referred to paediatric services. See Table 3.1 for a guide to understanding weight.

 Table 3.1 Guide to weight patterns and plotting

Weight

- Newborn infants lose up to 10 per cent of their birth weight within the first few days of life with weight gain commencing at three to five days. Weight is usually regained by two weeks.

- Feeds should be calculated on birth weight until this has been regained – after then, generally calculations are on *current* weight.

- Well term infants should be weighed according to individual assessment/need.

- Length and head circumference are other growth parameters, which indicate skeletal and organ growth. Unlike weight, these parameters are not influenced by fluid changes and fat deposition, but are not routinely monitored in well infants.

Plotting

- Plot neonatal weight/height/head circumference on recommended growth/centile chart. Birth is day 0.

- There are various charts depending on the gestation infants are born at (term, preterm or those requiring close monitoring).

- Royal College of Paediatrics and Child Health (RCPCH) growth charts, based on World Health Organization (WHO) Child Growth Standards, describe the optimal growth for healthy, breastfed children; they were updated in 2018 (Norris et al, 2018).

Table 3.1 (cont.)

- No line exists for the first two weeks to allow for the normal weight loss.
- If there is significant weight loss or the neonate is still below birth weight at two weeks, calculate the percentage weight loss.
- Weight loss of 10 per cent or more needs careful assessment: this can indicate dehydration.
- Monitoring of weight over time is important (observe the centile corresponding with the measured weight and the progression thereafter).
- Infants in the neonatal unit commonly lose weight and change/drop centiles if they spend a significant amount of time sick and in hospital (see Chapter 14).

(RCPCH, 2009)

Growth charts

Growth charts are used to monitor growth throughout childhood and provide information regarding rate of growth for weight, length and head circumference. Length and head circumference provide an indication of skeletal and organ growth, while weight is impacted by fluid change. Effective use of, and accurate plotting on, growth charts ensures that the child's growth is steady (RCPCH, 2009). An example of a growth chart is provided in Figure 3.1 and Table 3.2 summarises the recommended procedure for measuring weight (RCPCH, 2023). Within the UK, UK-WHO growth monitoring charts are utilised to regularly monitor growth both within acute and community settings. The guidance regarding frequency of monitoring will be determined by local guidance. Within the Personal Child Health Record ('red book'), there are growth monitoring charts, which do not replace any growth monitoring within acute settings. It is important to utilise the correct chart for the gender of the infant.

 There are fact sheets provided by RCPCH to support learning; written in 2009, they remain relevant and are hosted on their current website.

For preterm neonates and those requiring more frequent monitoring, there is the 'Neonatal and close monitoring growth chart' – see Chapter 14.

 Stop and think

It is important to refer to guidelines to avoid plotting errors; for example, age errors are a common source of mistakes.

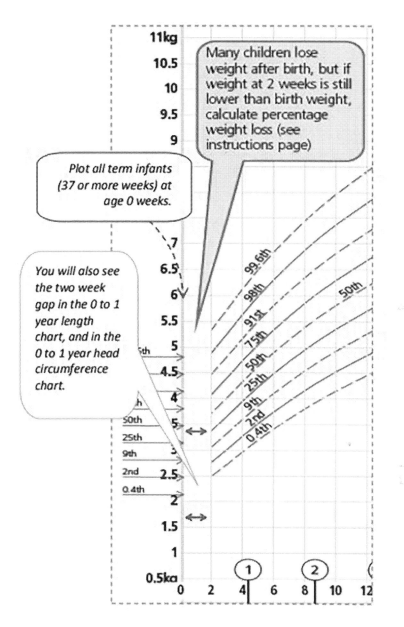

Figure 3.1 Example of a growth chart

© 2009 Royal College of Paediatrics and Child Health

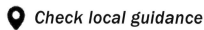

Check local guidance

Observe local guidance on agreed procedures for monitoring weight.

Table 3.2 Weight measurement

All measurers should be trained.
Weighing: • Use only class III electronic scales.   • Weigh babies naked.
Head circumference: • Use narrow paper or plastic tape round the widest part of the head.   • Best practice is to take an average of three measurements.
Length (up to age two):   • Proper equipment is essential (length board or mat).   • Nappy removed.   • Best practice is to take an average of three measurements.

Plotting summary
 • Record measurement and date in ink.
 • Plot in pencil.
 • Centile describes the percentage expected to be below that line.
 • A child is:
     – on a centile if within a quarter space of line;
     – between the two centiles if not.
 • A centile space is the distance between two centile lines.

(RCPCH, 2009)

Personal Child Health Record (red book)

Babies are issued with a Personal Child Health Record (PCHR) at birth, which is a national standard for recording growth, development and preventative health services. The record aims to improve continuity of communication with and between families and professionals. Currently, there is a pilot scheme for an electronic version with proposed benefits related to information sharing and accessibility (NHS Digital, 2023).

DEVELOPMENT

Babies are born with a range of reflexes (involuntary movements); examples are given in Table 3.3. These 'primary' reflexes gradually disappear as the baby grows and develops, while others, important for actions such as sitting and walking, prevail. Assessing for the presence of normal reflexes helps to identify that the brain and nervous system are functioning normally. It is also important to check that these are symmetrical.

⊞ Table 3.3 Normal newborn reflexes

Moro reflex – when the head is extended suddenly, the arms will both firstly extend with the hands and fingers fanned out, and then flex towards the body. Disappears at three to four months.
Grasp reflex – flexion of the fingers when an item is placed into the palm (palmar grasp). Also evident in the foot (plantar grasp). Palmar grasps disappear at around three months and plantar at eight months.
Babinski reflex – when the sole of the foot is firmly stroked, the big toe hyperextends and the rest of the toes fan out. Disappears by one year of age.
Rooting reflex – if the cheek is touched on one side the baby will turn their face towards that side and open the mouth. Disappears at around three to four months but may persist up to one year.
Sucking reflex – baby will automatically suck something placed in the mouth, such as a nipple or teat. Persists throughout infancy.
Stepping reflex – when held upright, with the soles of the feet touching a surface, the baby will lift their legs in a 'stepping' movement. Duration varies between individuals.
Asymmetrical tonic-neck reflex – when the baby is lying supine with their head facing in one direction, their arm will stretch out on that same side and the opposite arm flexes – sometimes known as the 'fencing reflex'. Disappears at three to four months (when the body is positioned symmetrically).

(NeuroRestart, 2023)

DEVELOPMENTAL INFLUENCES

Recently, increasing focus has been placed on how much of an impact an individual's experiences during the antenatal period, and within the first months of life, can have on their health and well-being throughout their lifespan. This is an important time with regard to development because the brain undergoes a period of huge evolution within the first year of life, with more than a million new neural connections being formed every second (HM Government, 2021). Initially, sensory pathways are laid down to support core functions such as hearing and vision before language and other higher cognitive functions then progress. Various factors influence development in early life (Figure 3.2).

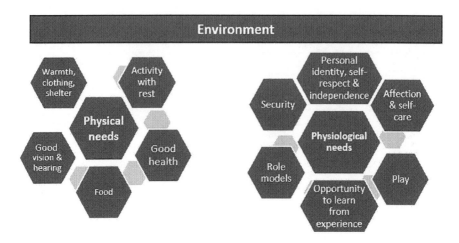

Figure 3.2 Physical and psychological needs and development

For infants to grow and reach their full developmental potential, it is important that their physical and psychosocial needs are met.

> *For children to meet their full potential, the environment optimal development, the environment must meet their needs within both domains.*
> (Lissauer and Claydon, 2018, p 28)

Lissauer and Claydon (2018) suggest that development can be considered in relation to four functional areas:

○ gross motor;

○ vision and fine motor;

○ hearing, speech and language;

○ social, emotional and behavioural.

Elements have been grouped together where they rely on each other – for example, development of speech and language relies on adequate hearing. Development occurs in a sequential manner, although there are variations in when skills are attained. Milestones (Table 3.4) are generally discussed in relation to the *median* age at which they are demonstrated (the 'middle' of the usual age range). It is also, however, important to be aware of '*limit ages*', by which time demonstration of a given skill would be expected, and investigations undertaken if this is not the case.

⊞ Table 3.4 Developmental milestones: expectations within the first year of life

---

Although many aspects of development occur after the neonatal period, big changes occur within the first 28 days.

By the end of their first month, most infants will:

- visually fix on and follow an object;
- make jerky, quivering arm movements;
- bring hands near face and keep hands in tight fists;
- move head from side to side while lying on stomach;
- focus on objects 20–25 cm away;
- prefer human faces and black-and-white or high-contrast patterns;
- turn towards noises, recognise and be settled by familiar voices;
- respond (stop crying) to social contact and stimuli such as being picked up or talked to and will maintain eye contact and recognise faces when they are close.

By the end of their third month, most infants will:

- raise head and chest, stretch legs out and kick when lying on stomach;
- push down on legs when feet are placed on a firm surface;
- open and shut hands;
- bring hands to mouth and start using hands and eyes in co-ordination;
- grab and shake hand toys;
- recognise familiar objects and people at a distance;
- begin to babble and to imitate some sounds;
- smile at the sound of parents'/primary caregivers' voices.

By the end of their seventh month, most infants will:

- roll over both ways and sit up;
- reach for objects and transfer objects from one hand to the other;
- develop full-colour vision and mature distance vision;
- respond to own name;
- babble chains of consonants;
- distinguish emotions by tone of voice;
- explore objects with hands and mouth;
- enjoy playing peek-a-boo.

By their first birthday, most infants will:

- sit without assistance;
- get into hands-and-knees position/may crawl/may pull self up to stand;

→

Table 3.4 (cont.)

- walk holding onto furniture, and possibly a few steps without support;

- use pincer grasp (thumb and forefinger);

- say '*dada*' and '*mama*' and try to imitate words;

- respond to '*no*' and simple verbal requests;

- explore objects in many ways (shaking, banging, throwing, dropping);

- begin to use objects correctly (drinking from cup, brushing hair);

- find hidden objects easily;

- look at correct picture when an image is named.

(March of Dimes, 2023)

 Stop and think

All infants are individuals and will have different developmental milestones in relation to timing. Individual variations must be considered.

 See the web companion for a glossary specific to this chapter.

 Check local variations and guidance alert

The space below can be used to record any notes or local variations and practice points specific to your own unit.

REFERENCES

British Nutrition Foundation, Sanders, T A B and Stannerin, S (2013) Normal Growth and Development. In *Nutrition and Development: Short- and Long-Term Consequences for Health* (pp 13–27). Chichester: Wiley-Blackwell.

HM Government (2021) *The Best Start for Life: A Vision for the 1,001 Critical Days*. London: HM Stationery Office.

Lissauer, T and Claydon, W (2018) *Illustrated Textbook of Paediatrics*. 5th ed. Oxford: Elsevier.

March of Dimes (2023) Developmental Milestones for Baby. [online] Available at: www.marchofdimes.org/find-support/topics/parenthood/developmental-milestones-baby (accessed 1 November 2023).

National Institute for Health and Care Excellence (NICE) (2017) Faltering Growth: Recognition and Management of Faltering Growth in Children. NICE Guideline [NG75]. [online] Available at: www.nice.org.uk/guidance/ng75 (accessed 1 November 2023).

NeuroRestart (2023) Primitive Reflexes. [online] Available at: www.neurorestart.co.uk/primitive-reflexes (accessed 1 November 2023).

NHS Digital (2023) Digital Child Health. [online] Available at: https://digital.nhs.uk/services/digital-child-health (accessed 1 November 2023).

Norris, T, Seaton, S E, Manktelow, B N et al (2018) Updated Birth Weight Centiles for England and Wales. *Archives of Disease in Childhood – Fetal and Neonatal Edition*, 103: F577–F582.

Royal College of Paediatrics and Child Health (RCPCH) (2009) *Measuring and Plotting: Fact Sheet 3*. [online] Available at: www.rcpch.ac.uk/sites/default/files/Measuring_and_plotting_advice.pdf (accessed 1 November 2023).

Royal College of Paediatrics and Child Health (RCPCH) (2023) UK-WHO Growth Charts – Guidance for Health Professionals. [online] Available at: www.rcpch.ac.uk/resources/uk-who-growth-charts-guidance-health-professionals (accessed 1 November 2023).

Toro-Ramos, T, Paley, C, Pi-Sunyer, F X and Gallagher, D (2015) Body Composition during Fetal Development and Infancy through the Age of 5 Years. *European Journal of Clinical Nutrition*, 69(12): 1279–89.

4 Assessment and screening of the healthy neonate

Julia Petty

INTRODUCTION

Assessment is an essential skill for any health professional working with neonates, which then forms the basis of any decision and subsequent intervention. It is important to ascertain and understand what normal assessment criteria are, so that any deviations can be noted and appropriate intervention undertaken. Assessment should be individualised to the specific neonate, situation or condition, holistically considering all systems including the family and psychosocial needs. This section focuses on assessment of the healthy term neonate (Tables 4.1 to 4.4) at birth and thereafter, including screening (Figure 4.1, Tables 4.5 to 4.7).

Chapter learning objectives

By the end of this chapter you will:

✓ have gained an overview and understanding of the key principles of assessment relating to the 'expected' norms for a healthy term neonate.

✓ be able to explain methods used for routine neonatal screening.

Critical thinking points

- Consider how you would assess whether a neonate is 'healthy' or not.

- What are key factors that would determine the sound health and well-being of a neonate?

Related topics: Assessment is a vital component of *any* aspect of care within this book. Assessment in the clinical setting (eg within the neonatal unit and hospital) is covered in Part 2, Chapter 10.

ASSESSMENT OF THE HEALTHY NEONATE AT BIRTH

Most neonates are born at term gestation (37 to 41 weeks) and are healthy. However, assessment is necessitated to ensure that any events during pregnancy and/or birth have not affected the growing infant in any adverse way and to highlight any reason for further attention.

Table 4.1 Assessment of the newborn baby at delivery

Sign	Score 0	Score 1	Score 2
Heart rate	Nil	<100	>100
Respiratory effort	Absent	Gasping or irregular	Regular or crying
Muscle tone	Flaccid	Some tone	Active
Response to stimulation	None	Grimace	Cry or cough
Colour	White	Blue	Pink centrally

For 'Apgar' scoring, score 0, 1 or 2 for each sign to ascertain a total score between 0 and 10. Take this at 1, 5 and 10 minutes of age. Consider the Apgar score along with information in Table 4.2. Assessment will determine subsequent management, if necessary.

 Stop and think

The five components that make up the traditional 'Apgar score' give practitioners a picture of whether the transition from intrauterine to extra-uterine life has gone smoothly or if there is a cause for any concern, even if a formal 'score' is not assigned.

Table 4.2 Assessment of the healthy neonate at birth and thereafter: additional considerations

- Record the Apgar score routinely at one and five minutes for all births.
- Record the time from birth to the onset of regular respirations.
- Umbilical cord care at birth: if the baby is 'well', delay cord clamping for one minute and give to parents for skin-to-skin holding. Ensure that a second clamp for double-clamping of the cord is available in all birth settings.
- Encourage skin-to-skin contact between parent and baby as soon as possible.
- To keep the baby warm and dry, cover them with a blanket or towel while maintaining skin-to-skin contact.
- Avoid separation of a mother and her baby during the first hour post-birth for the undertaking of routine postnatal procedures, for example, weighing, measuring and bathing, unless these activities are requested by the woman and/or medical staff or are necessary for immediate care.
- Encourage breastfeeding as soon as possible after the birth, ideally within one hour.
- Record head circumference, body temperature and birth weight soon after one hour.
- Undertake an initial examination/assessment to detect any major physical abnormalities and to identify any problems that require referral (➡ see Chapter 10 for further detail).
- At each postnatal contact, ask parents if they have any concerns about their baby's general well-being, feeding or development. Review the feeding history and assess the baby's health, including general concerns, physical inspection and observation. If there are any concerns, take appropriate further action.
- Be aware that if the baby has not passed meconium within 24 hours of birth, this may indicate a serious disorder and require medical advice.
- Conduct a complete examination of the baby within 72 hours of the birth.
- At six to eight weeks, assess the baby's social smiling and visual fixing and following.
- Measure weight and head circumference of the baby in the first week and at around eight weeks, and at other times, but only if there are concerns. Plot the results on the growth chart.
- Blood spot screening is undertaken at day 5, in line with the relevant newborn blood spot screening programme (➡ see Table 4.5) and specific country guidance (timelines may vary).
- Hearing screening is undertaken within six weeks, in line with the NHS newborn hearing screening programme (➡ see Table 4.6).
- Another complete examination of the baby at six to eight weeks after the birth is undertaken (Public Health England, 2013) (➡ see Table 4.7).
- Ensure that any examination of the baby is undertaken with parental consent.

(Adapted from NICE, 2017, 2021)

A SYSTEMATIC APPROACH TO ASSESSMENT AFTER BIRTH

A systems-based approach can be used to assess the healthy neonate in order to establish and ascertain expected normal features, that is, those not warranting referral or concern.

⊞ Table 4.3 Clinical assessment of the neonate

System	Normal/expected assessment criteria
Airway and breathing (respiratory)	Effortless breathing which may be periodic, normal rate, bilateral chest movement, quiet chest sounds, no oxygen requirement and oxygen saturations within normal range (see Table 4.4). Skin colour should be assessed in line with the neonate's skin tone and ethnicity.
Cardiovascular	Adequate heart rate/pulse and mean blood pressure (MBP) (see Table 4.4), capillary refill of less than 3 seconds and urine output of at least 1 ml/kg/hour. Mucous membranes (rather than skin) should be pink in colour, the skin should be warm, pulses palpable and the heart rate within normal limits.
Developmental/ behavioural and stress	No presence of pain or distress. Neonate is positioned appropriately – flexed limbs in mid-line, appears comfortable, relaxed and able to sleep for long periods.
Environmental/ thermal control	Normal body temperature (36.5–37.2 degrees Celsius) and appropriate environmental temperature according to age and gestation and birth weight.
Fluid status and balance	Adequate systemic perfusion and urine output (see above), normal/palpable fontanelles, palpable peripheral pulses, good skin turgor, normal blood sodium levels, specific gravity of urine 1.010–1.020, weight gain appropriate for age and equal fluid balance (in and out), ascertained by a hydration assessment.
Gastro-intestinal and nutritional status	Soft, non-tender abdomen, bowel sounds, nil/minimal regurgitation of feed from stomach which is clear mucous, bowels open and normal stool, no vomiting and tolerance of feeds if applicable.
The 3 Hs (metabolic adaptation)	Able to maintain adequate oxygenation, body temperature and blood glucose. For information on oxygenation and body temperature, see Table 4.4. Blood glucose should be >2.6 mmol/L in the first few hours, then 4–6 mmol/L thereafter.
Immunological	Signs of infection, such as a pyrexia, are not evident.

Table 4.3 (cont.)

System	Normal/expected assessment criteria
Jaundice (hepatic)	Physiological jaundice, due to liver immaturity, is common: observe for signs of clinical jaundice/yellow skin on blanching and sclera of eyes. Serum or transcutaneous bilirubin is below treatment threshold (see Chapter 8 for thresholds).
Muscular-skeletal	Presence of well-toned and flexed posture with spontaneous movements. Legs able to adduct and abduct and move without 'clicking' or hindrance within the hip joint.
Neurological and sensory	Response to stimuli, such as pain, is present at birth. Neonate is alert, wakes when hungry and can feed. Normal/present reflexes are exhibited according to gestation and age.
Skin and general appearance	Expected skin appearance for gestation, eg well formed in term neonates, good skin integrity with no or minimal dryness or flaking. Expected skin colour and presentation for skin tone/ethnicity – eg Mongolian blue spot may be present at the top of buttocks in Asian and Black babies. No excoriation present or signs of jaundice. Umbilical area is clean and dry. Intravenous (IV) access sites, if present, should appear healthy with no signs of leakage or interstitial infiltration.

➡ The focus of the above guide is physical assessment. Family adjustment to birth and parenting, along with assessment of psychosocial needs, is covered in detail in Chapter 6.

(Adapted from Petty, 2011; McDonald and Kaiser, 2020; Lomax, 2021)

For '*normal*' ranges and parameters for vital signs, refer to Table 4.4.

 Stop and think

While assessment, as applied to the *systems*, can help impart a systematic structure to the process, it should be considered within a holistic perspective. For example, any vital sign must be interpreted according to the individual neonate's condition and alongside clinical assessment.

EXPECTED VITAL SIGNS

Taking observations of key vital signs is a fundamental assessment skill in neonatal care. It is important that neonatal norms are understood so that any deviation from this is identified. Table 4.4 outlines the normal parameters across the developmental spectrum.

 Table 4.4 An information guide to neonatal specific parameters and values

Heart rate: beats per minute (bpm)

Age	Awake	Sleeping
Neonate (preterm)	100–200	120–180
Neonate (term)	100–180	80–160
Infant	100–160	75–160
Toddler	80–110	60–90
Preschooler	70–110	60–90
School	65–110	60–90

Blood pressure (mmHg)

Age	Systolic	Diastolic
Birth (12 hr, <1 kg)	39–59	16–36
Birth (12 hr, 3 kg)	50–70	24–45
Neonate (96 hr)	60–90	20–60
Infant (6 month)	87–105	53–66
Toddler (2 year)	95–105	53–66
School age	97–112	57–71
Adult	112–128	66–80

NB: In neonates, it is vital to consider the **mean arterial blood pressure (MABP)**. As a *general* guide, the gestational age in weeks should correspond with mean BP (eg a baby born at 40 weeks should have a MABP of 40 mmHg).

→

Table 4.4 (cont.)

Respiratory rates:	Breaths per minute (bpm)
Preterm	40–80
Term neonates	30–70
Infants	30–60
Toddlers	24–40
Preschool	22–34
School/adult	18–30

Temperature	(degrees Celsius)
Central (axilla)	36.6–37.2
Abdominal (probe)	36.6–37.2 (preterm), 35.5–36.5 (term)
Peripheral (foot)	34.6–36.2
Core-toe temperature gap	less than 2 degrees Celsius

Oxygen saturation (SpO$_2$)	
95–100%	

Perfusion	
Capillary refill time	less than 3 seconds (RCN, 2017)
Urine output	minimum of 1 ml/kg/hour

Circulating blood volume	
Neonates	85–90 ml/kg
Infants	75–80 ml/kg
Children	70–75 ml/kg
Adults	65–70 ml/kg

Tidal volumes (air volume per respiratory cycle)	
Neonates	4–6 ml/kg
Children	6–10 ml/kg

Blood glucose	
After transition at birth >2.5 mmol/L at birth (BAPM, 2017)	
4–6 mmol/L, after the newborn period and in children/adults.	

(Adapted from RCN, 2017; Lapum et al, 2015)

Stop and think

Understanding the normal range of vital signs is important to serve as a baseline with which to compare assessed parameters and decide whether these require attention. All values are *averages* and should serve as a guideline in conjunction with the overall assessment of the individual neonate.

SCREENING IN THE NEONATE

Screening is an important area of healthcare and is necessary for the early identification of the risk of a neonate having certain disease(s); this enables timely and appropriate action to be taken, following a diagnosis. Antenatal screening via scanning or blood testing may identify neonates at risk even prior to delivery. Such tests include screening for infectious diseases (hepatitis B, HIV and syphilis), inherited conditions (sickle cell, thalassaemia and other haemoglobin disorders), chromosomal conditions such as Down's, Edwards's and Patau's syndromes, and physical anomalies at the 20-week scan. Tables 4.5 to 4.7 provide an overview to guide three main areas of screening in the neonatal period: bloodspot screening, hearing screening and examination of the newborn, respectively. The NHS National Screening Committee makes appropriate recommendations for all areas of screening including both antenatal and postnatal tests.

 Stop and think

Screening identifies a risk of having or developing a disease. It is *not* a diagnosis.

▦ Table 4.5 Neonatal blood spot screening

Screening overview

How?	Why?
• Follow the steps laid out in the national guidance (Public Health England, 2021).	The following six recessive genetic, metabolic disorders are screened for:
• The routine blood spot sample (four spots) should be taken on day 5 for all babies. Day of birth is day 0.	• phenylketonuria (PKU) • medium chain acyl coenzyme A dehydrogenase deficiency (MCADD);

Table 4.5 (cont.)

Screening overview

How?	Why?
• In exceptions, a sample can be taken between day 5 and day 8.	• maple syrup urine disease (MSUD);
• Ensure parents have access to the pre-screening booklet at least 24 hours before taking the sample.	• isovaleric acidaemia (IVA); • glutaric aciduria type 1 (GA1);
• Clean the heel, wash hands thoroughly and ensure the infant is comfortable.	• homocystinuria (HCU). In addition, the following conditions are also screened for:
• Obtain the sample using an age-appropriate automated incision device, not a manual lancet. See Figure 4.1 for the preferred puncture sites. Allow the heel to hang down to assist blood flow. The skin puncture must be no deeper than 2 mm.	• sickle cell disease; • cystic fibrosis (CF); • congenital hypothyroidism; • surveillance for maternal human immune deficiency virus (HIV) (anonymous testing, not individual diagnosis).
• Obtain four blood spots on the blood spot card, completed with the infant's details.	Metabolic diseases such as PKU and congenital hypothyroidism are conditions, which, if untreated, can result in significant developmental delay.
• Ensure consent is recorded as well as the actual test in the relevant documentation according to specific country guidance or medical notes.	

For full information on national guidance, see Public Health England (2021).

 Stop and think

All screening should be explained to the parents, including the reasons for performing it and any subsequent actions that may be required.

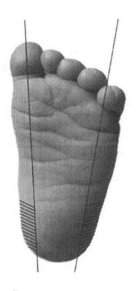
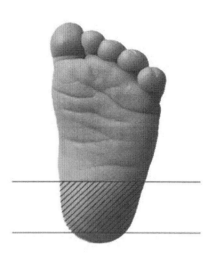

 Figure 4.1 Preferred sites for heel prick blood sampling in a neonate (Public Health England, 2021)

Table 4.6 Summary of neonatal hearing screening

How?	Why?
• ALL neonates should have hearing screening prior to discharge from hospital OR arranged in the community within six weeks (post-term corrected age). • The screen uses two tests called the otoacoustic emissions test (OAE) and the automated auditory brainstem response test (AABR). Both tests are painless.	• The aim is to identify any hearing loss that could go on to affect language acquisition in the developing infant/child. In turn, intervention is given as soon as possible to prevent a delay in this vital area of development. • Neonates who do not show strong responses will be referred for a full diagnostic assessment.

For full information on national guidance, see Public Health England (2016).

🖐 *Stop and think*

The implications of hearing loss in the at-risk neonate must be considered in line with future sensory outcomes.

Table 4.7 Checklist for physical examination of the neonate

When?	Why?
Physical examination should take place at the following stages: • at birth; • within the first 24 hours; • at 72 hours; • at 6 weeks.	To detect any conditions, anomalies or dysmorphic features that may need early treatment and referral.

How? A full examination should include...

- Appearance, including skin colour, breathing, behaviour, activity and posture.
- Head (including fontanelles), face, nose, mouth (including palate), ears, neck and general symmetry of head and facial features.
- Eyes: opacities, red reflex and colour of sclera.
- Neck and clavicles, limbs, hands, feet and digits; assessment of proportions and symmetry.
- Heart: position, heart rate, rhythm and sounds, murmurs and femoral pulse volume.
- Lungs: respiratory effort, rate and lung sounds.
- Abdomen: assessment of shape; palpation to identify any organomegaly; checking of condition of the umbilical cord.
- Genitalia and anus: completeness and patency and undescended testes in boys.
- Spine: inspection and palpation of bony structures; checking of skin integrity.
- Skin: assessment of colour and texture as well as any birthmarks or rashes.
- Central nervous system: muscle tone, behaviour, movements and posture; checking of newborn reflexes, but only if concerned.
- Hips: symmetry of the limbs, Barlow and Ortolani's manoeuvres.
- Cry: assessment of sound.
- Weight: document.

(Full guidance: Public Health England (2013); Jones (2019); Lomax (2011))

 Stop and think

The full guidance should be referred to for any screening. The above offers a summary and short synopsis only as an overview.

Standard precautions alert

Wash hands thoroughly before and after examining/handling infants for assessment purposes.

 See the web companion for a glossary specific to this chapter.

 Check local variations and guidance alert

The space below can be used to record any notes or local variations and practice points specific to your own unit.

REFERENCES

British Association of Perinatal Medicine (BAPM) (2017) Identification and Management of Neonatal Hypoglycaemia in the Full-Term Infant: A BAPM Framework for Practice. [online] Available at: www.bapm.org/resources/40-identification-and-management-of-neonatal-hypoglycaemia-in-the-full-term-infant-2017 (accessed 31 October 2023).

Jones, T (ed) (2019) *The Student Guide to the Newborn Infant Physical Examination*. Oxford: Routledge.

Lapum, J I, Verkuyl, M, Garcia, W, St-Amant, C and Tan, A (2015) *Vital Sign Measurement Across the Lifespan*. 1st ed. [online] Available at: https://pressbooks.library.ryerson.ca/vitalsign (accessed 31 October 2023).

Lomax, A (ed) (2011) *Examination of the Newborn: An Evidence Based Guide*. 3rd ed. Oxford: Wiley-Blackwell.

McDonald, L and Kaiser, L (2020) Assessment of the Neonate. In Boxwell, G, Petty, J and Kaiser, L (eds) *Neonatal Intensive Care Nursing*. 3rd ed (Chapter 2). Oxford: Routledge.

National Institute for Health and Care Excellence (NICE) (2017) Intrapartum Care for Healthy Women and Babies. Clinical Guideline [CG190]. [online] Available at: www.nice.org.uk/guidance/cg190 (accessed 31 October 2023).

National Institute for Health and Care Excellent (NICE) (2021) Postnatal Care NICE Guideline. Clinical Guideline [NG194]. [online] Available at: www.nice.org.uk/guidance/ng194 (accessed 31 October 2023).

Petty, J (2011) Fact Sheet; Neonatal Biology – An Overview Parts 1, 2 & 3. *Journal of Neonatal Nursing*, 17(2–4): 128–31.

Public Health England (2013) Newborn and Infant Physical Examination (NIPE) Screening: Programme Overview. [online] Available at: www.gov.uk/guidance/newborn-and-infant-physical-examination-screening-programme-overview (accessed 31 October 2023).

Public Health England (2016) Newborn Hearing Screening Programme. [online] Available at: www.gov.uk/guidance/newborn-hearing-screening-programme-overview (accessed 31 October 2023).

Public Health England (2021) Newborn Blood Spot Sampling Guidelines: Quick Reference Guide. [online] Available at: www.gov.uk/government/publications/newborn-blood-spot-screening-sampling-guidelines/quick-reference-guide (accessed 31 October 2023).

Royal College of Nursing (RCN) (2017) *Standards for Assessing, Measuring and Monitoring Vital Signs in Infants, Children and Young People. RCN Guidance for Nurses Working with Children and Young People*. [online] Available at: www.rcn.org.uk/professional-development/publications/pub-005942 (accessed 31 October 2023).

5 Important practices for neonatal health

Sheila Roberts

INTRODUCTION

From the moment a baby is born they become an individual with their own needs, their own characteristics and their own family. Despite the uniqueness of all babies, they all have fundamental needs in the early months of life that are primarily the same regardless of race or culture: these are a need to be comforted, the need for adequate nutrition and the need to be protected from harm. When these fundamental needs are met, the infant has the maximum opportunity to grow and thrive both physically and emotionally. This chapter looks at some of the principles that aim to meet the fundamental needs of an infant in relation to comfort and pain management, infection prevention and feeding (Figure 5.1; Tables 5.1 to 5.3).

Chapter learning objectives

By the end of this chapter you will:

✓ be able to recognise the importance of providing comfort to an infant and consider how this may be achieved;

✓ have some understanding of the nutritional needs of, and infection prevention methods for, an infant.

Critical thinking points

- Consider how you can recognise the distress signals of a young infant and how to provide the necessary comfort.

- Consider how you would meet the nutritional requirements and sound infection control for a range of infants you meet in clinical practice.

See also Chapter 8 for feeding and infection and Chapter 9 for pain management, relating to the sick and premature neonate in the neonatal unit.

 See the web companion for supplementary information on the above topics.

COMFORT AND WELL-BEING

Comfort

Comfort and well-being are important for everyone and no less so for the neonate and infant. Comfort comes in various forms.

○ Touch is a fundamental human requirement and helps to build a strong bond between infant and parents. Touch, such as a hug, produces serotonin, primarily in the intestine, which then acts as a neurotransmitter, and oxytocin, produced in the hypothalamus and released by the posterior pituitary. Both hormones are associated with happiness and well-being (Ellingsen et al, 2016).

○ Kangaroo care or skin-to-skin contact (SSC) is known to have many benefits in the immediate post-delivery period (Unicef, 2024). It helps the newborn adjust to their new surroundings in a calm, comforting manner. It helps to stabilise vital signs, including blood sugar levels while providing warmth and comfort. SSC also provides a strong bond for both parents (see Chapter 6), encourages lactation for the mother and more successful breastfeeding, which in turn positively affects the neonate's weight gain. SSC can be continued beyond the initial newborn period to lower stress levels, encourage sleep and enhance overall comfort for the infant and parent. There is some evidence that suggests SSC aids parent–infant attachment and has a positive influence on neurodevelopment in premature infants (see Chapters 6 and 9).

○ Swaddling a newborn in a lightweight blanket can provide comfort and encourage sleep. However, a swaddled infant may cry less and visual feeding cues, such as fists to mouth, are obscured; this can have a negative effect on establishing and maintaining breastfeeding.

○ 'Baby massage' is a known technique to promote comfort and reduce irritability in an infant. Parents can be encouraged to engage in baby massage, starting with gentle stroking or nurturing touch from newborn and building to full baby massage after a few weeks. Baby massage increases bonding and helps the infant to feel nurtured and loved (International Association of Infant Massage, 2023).

Stop and think

Infants who are swaddled immediately after birth may have a delay in initial breastfeeding and may be less successful at establishing breast-feeding. This results in a reduced intake of breast milk and greater weight loss compared to unswaddled babies (Dixley and Ball, 2023).

Pain

Although neonates and infants have immature nervous systems, they do feel pain and they have a right for that pain to be identified and treated. Signs that infants may be in pain are summarised in Table 5.1.

Table 5.1 Infant pain cues

Crying	Infants cry for various reasons, but when in pain this may be prolonged, and the pitch of the cry may be higher.
Facial expressions	Infants in pain are likely to squeeze their eyes tightly shut and have furrowed brows, with a deepening of the nasolabial furrow and mouth open. Their chin may quiver.
Muscle tension	It is likely that an infant in pain will tense their muscles in either a pulling in motion or extended position – called flailing.
Movement	This will depend on the age and energy level of the infant; they may squirm and vigorously move their arms and legs or may be quite still.
Sleep	An infant in pain is likely to be irritable and have disturbed sleep.
Feeding	An infant in pain is likely to be reluctant with feeds or just take small amounts.
Physiological factors	The heart rate will generally increase when an infant is in pain, and breathing may become faster and shallow. Blood pressure increases, while oxygen saturations decrease.

Pain assessment

There are a variety of formal pain assessment tools available for assessing pain in a neonate and infant.

- o **FLACC** – **F**acial expression, **L**eg movement, **A**ctivity, **C**ry and **C**onsolability (Merkel et al, 1997), where each indicator is scored on a 0–2 scale, giving a total of between 0 (no pain) and 10 (extreme pain). Although well established and straightforward to use, there is some subjectivity in relation to consolability.

- o **CRIES** – **C**ry, **R**equires oxygen to maintain oxygen saturations above 95%, **I**ncreased vital signs, **E**xpressions and **S**leeplessness (Krechel and Bildner, 1995). This tool is suitable to use from birth within a clinical setting where vital signs and oxygen saturation can be measured. It is straightforward to use, but it is important to remember that changes in vital signs may be indicative of a range of factors.

- o **PIPP** – **P**remature **I**nfant **P**ain **P**rofile (Stevens et al, 2014, cited by Perry et al, 2018) is suitable for full-term neonates as well as premature infants. This tool measures on a scale of 0–3 and takes into consideration gestational age, behaviour (awake/active/asleep), heart rate, oxygen saturations, brow bulge, eye squeeze and nasolabial furrow.

- o **COMFORT** – this tool can be used for neonates in intensive care receiving ventilation (van Dijk et al, 2009, cited by Perry et al, 2018).

- o **NFCS** – the **N**eonatal **F**acial **C**oding **S**ystem is an anatomically based assessment of acute pain using ten different facial expressions and is suitable for premature infants up to about 18 months (Grunau and Craig, 1987).

 Stop and think

Always choose the most relevant pain assessment tool for the situation and be aware that changes in vital signs can be indicative of a range of factors.

 See the web companion site for examples of pain assessment tools – the PIPP and COMFORT scales (Perry et al, 2018).

Being aware of pain away from the clinical setting is equally important. Parents will quickly become tuned to their own infant and recognise the signs and symptoms relating to pain. This may be a combination of any of the above.

Pain management

Management of pain in the non-clinical setting will vary from infant to infant and family to family, but may include:

○ touch such as cuddling, kangaroo care or stroking the infant, specifically stroking the head can be comforting;

○ talking quietly and gently, providing reassurance;

○ taking the infant to a quiet area, away from additional stimulation such as noise and bright lights;

○ swaddling the infant;

○ offering a feed or, if used, a pacifier;

○ changing the infant's nappy to ensure comfort;

○ analgesia can be given – paracetamol liquid can be used from one month of age and ibuprofen from three months of age.

 Stop and think

Paracetamol and ibuprofen must be given in accordance with the manufacturer's guidance and based on the infant's age and weight. Parents need to be aware to seek medical advice if the infant is not comforted and the pain continues.

INFECTION PREVENTION

The key principles of hand hygiene, personal protective equipment and universal precautions within a clinical setting are not necessarily relevant within the home setting. However, it is important that neonates and infants are protected as far as possible from infection. Key principles include:

○ hygiene;

○ vaccinations.

Hygiene

Hand hygiene, even at home, remains the key principle for protecting a young infant from infection and the rules for good hand hygiene should be reinforced. The importance of hand hygiene (Figure 5.1) is relevant to families but also anyone entering the house and in contact with the infant.

o   Wet hands under warm running water.

o   Soap.

o   Scrub all aspects of the hands; fingers and thumbs need to be thoroughly washed.

o   Rinse.

o   Dry with paper or other towel.

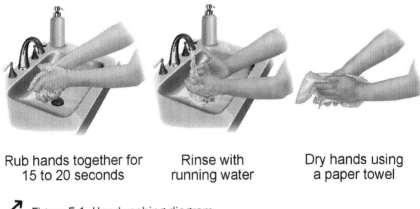

Rub hands together for   Rinse with   Dry hands using
    15 to 20 seconds   running water   a paper towel

↗ Figure 5.1 Handwashing diagram

General home hygiene includes the safe disposal of soiled nappies, the use of anti-bacterial cleaners on surfaces, especially in the kitchen and bathroom, and on baby equipment such as highchairs; bacteria can live on surfaces for up to 48 hours. Disposable tissues are more hygienic than cotton handkerchiefs and help to keep the home environment clean. Families should be encouraged to give up smoking; smoke lingers on furniture, clothes and in hair and will have a detrimental impact on an infant's health. Dropped pacifiers or bottles should be replaced with clean versions and not placed in the parent's mouth, which is known to contain numerous bacteria and viruses.

Good baby hygiene will also help to prevent infections. It is recommended that babies are not bathed for the first 24 hours as the vernix, a waxy white substance that coats a baby's skin before birth, acts as a natural moisturiser and may have anti-bacterial properties. After this, warm water is sufficient until the baby is about four to six weeks old when an unperfumed baby bath can be introduced. Particular attention needs to be given to skin fold areas to prevent soreness and potential infection. Regular changing of nappies prevents nappy rash, which if left untreated is not only uncomfortable but may lead to infection. Dental care is also important; the first teeth should erupt at about the age of six months and simple brushing along with good oral hygiene should commence at that point to prevent decay and cavities in the milk teeth and later in life.

Vaccinations

Vaccinations form an important aspect of an infant's general well-being and prevent ill-health. Healthcare professionals should use every opportunity to promote the importance of vaccinations to parents and carers. Infectious diseases are not only distressing for an infant but can cause lasting damage; for example, measles, while generally mild in most cases, can lead to encephalitis and brain damage. Where there is good uptake of the vaccinations, diseases can be eliminated, for example polio and diphtheria, or reduced, for example, measles and whooping cough. Table 5.2 provides an overview of the UK's immunisation schedule for infants up to one year of age.

⊞ Table 5.2 Immunisation schedule

Age of infant	Vaccine	Disease protected against
8 weeks	DtaP/IPV/Hib/HepB	Diphtheria, tetanus, pertussis (whooping cough), polio, Haemophilus influenzae type B, hepatitis B
	MenB	Meningococcal group B
	Rotavirus	Rotavirus-induced gastroenteritis
12 weeks	DtaP/IPV/Hib/HepB	Diphtheria, tetanus, pertussis (whooping cough), polio, Haemophilus influenzae type B, hepatitis B
	PCV – pneumococcal conjugate vaccine	Pneumococcal disease
	Rotavirus	Rotavirus-induced gastroenteritis
16 weeks	DtaP/IPV/Hib/HepB	Diphtheria, tetanus, pertussis (whooping cough), polio, Haemophilus influenzae type B, hepatitis B
	Men B	Meningococcal group B

→

Table 5.2 (cont.)

Age of infant	Vaccine	Disease protected against
1 year	Hib/Men C	Haemophilus influenzae type B, meningococcal group C
	PCV booster	Pneumococcal disease
	MMR	Measles, mumps and rubella (German measles)
	Men B booster	Meningococcal group B
Additional vaccines in specific population groups		
Older infants – from 2 years old	LAIV (Live attenuated influenza vaccine)	Influenza Given to high-risk groups
4 weeks	BCG (Bacillus Calmette-Guérin)	Tuberculosis (TB). Given to infants living in an area with a high TB incidence or infants with a parent or grandparent born in a high-incidence country.

(Gov.uk 2023)

NUTRITION

The period from birth to one year is one of rapid growth and development. To meet the demands of this growth, optimal nutrition is essential to the infant. Where the optimal nutritional needs are not met the infant will not thrive, which leads to health problems in the short and long term, even into adulthood. The healthy infant between birth and one year requires 100 kilocalories/kilogram of body weight/day. About half of this requirement is used for basal metabolism, with thermoregulation accounting for much of this requirement, along with feeding, digestion, absorption, storage and elimination also requiring a vast amount of energy, often up to 30–50 kcal/kg/day (Patel and Rouster, 2023). Optimal nutrition includes the requirement not only for adequate calories but also all food groups, macronutrients – protein, fats and carbohydrates – along with micro-nutrients and trace elements such as vitamins and iron.

Breastfeeding

The World Health Organization (2023) recommends exclusive breastfeeding for the first six months of life with the first feed taking place within an hour of birth. Ideally, breastfeeding should continue even after the introduction of weaning foods and should be the main source of nutrition up to one year of age. Breastfeeding has many benefits for the mother and the baby, including protection against infections, such as gastroenteritis. Breastfeeding is linked to a reduction in respiratory infections, including the development of asthma, a reduction in the potential to develop allergies and later in life a reduction in developing type 2 diabetes and obesity. Colostrum, the first milk to be produced, is thick and yellow in colour; it is high in protein and contains immunoglobulins that help to build the baby's immune system. Colostrum and/or breast milk has also been shown to have healing properties for conditions such as cradle cap, nappy rash and umbilical cord separation and can be beneficial for mothers with cracked nipples.

 Information box

Colostrum harvesting can take place from about 36 weeks' gestation; mothers are encouraged to express and safely store colostrum prior to their baby's delivery. This protein and immunoglobulin rich breast milk can be used should the baby have difficulties in establishing feeding in the initial newborn period or later if the baby becomes unwell.

 Stop and think

Midwives must be involved in the decision-making process prior to a pregnant woman commencing colostrum harvesting as there is a small chance it will initiate labour, especially if there is a history of premature births.

Formula feeding

Where breastfeeding is not possible or is not the parental choice, infants are fed on formula feeds. There are a range of formula milks available on the market and all must comply with the legalities with regard to production and composition of the feeds. Formula milk is primarily made from modified cow's milk and is either whey or casein protein dominant. Whey formulas are suitable from birth, whereas casein formulas are often marketed for the 'hungrier' baby as they require more complex digestion and may provide the baby with feelings of being full – there is however no scientific evidence to support this.

While breastfeeding is deemed best for baby in that it is nutritionally balanced to meet their requirements, the advantage of formula feeding is that it is possible to know exactly how much feed the baby has taken. See Table 5.3 for feed requirements and an example of the number of feeds a baby may require.

⊞ Table 5.3 Infant feeding

Age of baby	Feed requirement	Approximate timing of feeds
0–3 months	150 ml/kg/day	Every 3–4 hours
4–6 months	150 ml/kg/day	Every 4–6 hours
7–9 months	120 ml/kg/day – the baby will also now be having additional food	Probably four times a day
10–12 months	110 ml/kg/day, alongside additional food	Probably three times a day

 Stop and think

Cultural preferences should always be taken into account in relation to parental decisions including feeding choices. In addition, individualised care should also be highlighted here, for example neonates are individuals and may for a variety of reasons require changes to the above nutritional requirements as well as feeding methods.

Specialised infant formulas

There are a range of specialised formula feeds for babies with specific nutritional requirements such as:

o   preterm and low birthweight babies requiring additional calories;

o   thickened formulas as an anti-reflux feed;

o   lactose-free formulas;

o   soya-based formulas for cow's milk intolerance.

There is also a range of formula feeds available to meet the needs of babies with varying metabolic conditions; vegetarian, vegan and halal formula is also available.

 Stop and think

Another very important practice is the administration of vitamin K at birth to prevent vitamin K deficiency bleeding, given by an intramuscular injection (IM) or orally following discussion with a midwife.

IM vitamin K is given as a single dose at birth. Oral regimes must be repeated. Current guidance recommends 2 mg given at birth and again at one week of age (day 7). Babies who are exclusively formula fed require no further doses as artificial formula has synthetic vitamin K added. In exclusively breastfeeding infants, it is recommended that one further oral dose is given at one month of age (British National Formulary for Children (BNFC), 2024).

 ## *Standard precautions alert*

This chapter has emphasised the importance of good practice in relation to ensuring infection prevention measures are adhered to in order to avoid any risk to the infant in their first year.

 See the web companion for a glossary specific to this chapter.

 ## *Check local variations and guidance alert*

The space below can be used to record any notes or local variations and practice points specific to your own unit.

REFERENCES

Dixley, A and Ball, H L (2023) The Impact of Swaddling upon Breastfeeding: A Critical Review. *American Journal of Human Biology*, 35(6): e23878.

Ellingsen, D M, Leknes, S, Løseth, G, Wessberg, J and Olausson, H (2016) The Neurobiology Shaping Affective Touch: Expectation, Motivation, and Meaning in the Multisensory Context. *Frontiers in Psychology*, 6(6): 1–16.

Gov.uk (2023) Guidance: Complete Routine Immunisation Schedule from 1 September 2023. [online] Available at: www.gov.uk/government/publications/the-complete-routine-immunisation-schedule/the-complete-routine-immunisation-schedule-from-february-2022 (accessed 23 January 2024).

Grunau, R V E and Craig, K D (1987) Pain Expression in Neonates: Facial Action and Cry. *Pain*, 28: 395–410.

International Association of Infant Massage (2023) About Infant Massage. [online] Available at: www.iaim.org.uk/about-baby-massage (accessed 23 January 2024).

Krechel, S W and Bildner, J (1995) CRIES: A New Neonatal Postoperative Pain Measurement Score. Initial Testing of Validity and Reliability. *Pediatric Anesthesia*, 5: 53–61.

Merkel, S I, Voepel-Lewis, T, Shayevitz, J R and Malviya, S (1997) The FLACC: A Behavioral Scale for Scoring Postoperative Pain in Young Children. *Pediatric Nursing*, 23(3): 293–6.

Patel, J K and Rouster, A S (2023) Infant Nutrition Requirements and Options. In *StatPearls.* Treasure Island, FL: StatPearls Publishing.

Perry, M, Tan, Z, Chen, J, Weidig, T, Xu, W and Cong, X S (2018) Neonatal Pain: Perceptions and Current Practice. *Critical Care Nursing Clinics of North America*, 30(4): 549–61.

UNICEF (2024) Skin-to-skin Contact. [online] Available at: www.unicef.org.uk/babyfriendly/baby-friendly-resources/implementing-standards-resources/skin-to-skin-contact (accessed 23 January 2024).

World Health Organization (2023) Breastfeeding. [online] Available at: www.who.int/health-topics (accessed 1 November 2023).

6 Principles of family care

Laura Maguire and Jo Day

INTRODUCTION

The promotion of early bonding is vital to enhance the social and emotional development of the infant, building the foundations for relationships with others over their life course. There are a variety of benefits for both the infant and their family as well as strategies that can be utilised to support early bonding and facilitate healthy and secure attachments; some of these are explored in this chapter (Tables 6.1 to 6.6). Preferences relating to culture, ethnic background and religion should be always embraced and integrated into inclusive and equitable care when considering the family.

Chapter learning objectives

By the end of this chapter you will:

✓ understand why early bonding and secure attachment is fundamental to ensuring that children become happy, independent and resilient adults;

✓ be able to identify strategies to support and facilitate early bonding and secure attachment for the infant and their family.

Critical thinking points

- Identify potential barriers to early bonding and secure attachment and consider how you could overcome these in your practice.

- Consider how you could promote culturally appropriate strategies for early bonding to facilitate healthy and secure attachment.

 For specific family care in relation to the infant in the neonatal unit and at home after discharge from hospital, see Chapters 12 and 15.

See the web companion for supplementary information on family care, including a summary of inclusive neonatal nursing practice relating to families with individual protected characteristics (eg those from diverse ethnic backgrounds/minority ethnic groups, the LGBTQIA+ population and disabled and neurodiverse parents).

BONDING

Having a loving bond with a primary caregiver is vital for the infant as this facilitates brain development, including social, emotional and cognitive domains (Winston and Chicot, 2016). Bonding can be achieved using a variety of strategies (Table 6.1). Other simple strategies include cuddling, chatting and making eye contact. As brain development is substantive in these first months and years, these early experiences are crucial for successful positive long-term outcomes. Love, language and attention lead to the development of pathways that support memories and the formation of relationships (Winston and Chicot, 2016). Again, the culture and ethnicity of the parents should be considered for culturally appropriate care (Care Quality Commission, 2022).

⊞ Table 6.1 Strategies to support bonding

Strategy	Rationale	Evidence
Skin-to-skin	• Increases breastfeeding rates. • Facilitates stability of cardio-respiratory system. • Increases blood glucose levels. • Regulates stress, anxiety and psychological stress.	Moore et al (2016) Ionio et al (2021) Olsson et al (2017)
Reading	• Facilitates earlier speech development. • Soothing for infant. • Provides a structured activity to build parental confidence.	Brown et al (2017)
Singing	• Increase in postnatal bonding. • Reduction in incidence of crying episodes. • Reduction in episodes of infant colic. • Positive impact on maternal stress and neonatal behaviour.	Persico et al (2017)

Strategy	Rationale	Evidence
Cues and observational awareness	• Enables parents to observe the small daily changes in their infant. • Provides a focus in the early days. • Helps to build early bonds and enables parents to get to know their infant.	Olsson et al (2017)
Infant massage (from six weeks)	• Builds responsiveness between the infant and parents. • Improves weight gain, reduces unsettledness and improves sleep for infant. • Reduces depression and anxiety among parents. • Builds confidence and enjoyment of parenting. • Promotes bonding and closeness with the infant.	Vincente and Pereira (2021)
Well infant clinic	• Provides a community space to support new parents and their infants. • Gives an opportunity for information sharing to build confidence and promote a loving and gentle approach to parenting.	Winston and Chicot (2016)

Skin-to-skin care

Skin-to-skin contact (SSC, sometimes referred to as kangaroo care) was introduced in Chapter 5 and is an effective method to promote both early bonding and attachment. Parents should be encouraged to do this immediately after birth and it should continue throughout the early years of life. SSC has a positive effect on both the infant and parent and can regulate stress, anxiety and psychological stress (Ionio et al, 2021). It is important to remember that both parents can take part in SSC with there being benefits for main carers as well as the infant (Olsson et al, 2017). In a hospital setting, parents can be encouraged to place the infant on their chest, covered by a blanket or towel to keep the infant warm and to ensure the carers feel comfortable. On discharge, parents can spend time with their infant undertaking SSC for comfort, to help settle the infant, when feeding (either breast or bottle) and as a part of bath time or play time. Cultural preferences should always be taken into account for any care practice including SSC.

 Stop and think

Always follow sudden infant death syndrome (SIDS) guidance and be sure to share this information with parents. The Lullaby Trust provides up-to-date, evidence-based advice for professionals, parents and caregivers around reducing the risks of SIDS.

For skin-to-skin care relating to the infant in the neonatal unit, see Chapter 9.

PLAY AND COMMUNICATION

Play and communication are vital aspects of development and are crucial to good bonding and attachment relationships. Early play and communication can promote the development of pathways that create memories and support the development of healthy loving relationships. Suggested activities are shown in Table 6.2. Infants start to communicate from birth; encouraging parents to tune into these early communications is a key part of bonding. Learning what the infant's facial expressions may mean as well as noticing when the infant looks at them will help to build confidence and facilitate bonding (Harding et al, 2022). Infants who have their body language noticed and responded to feel safe and secure and may cry less.

 Table 6.2 Play and communication activities

These can include:

- reading;
- talking;
- singing;
- use of mirrors to look at self and the infant's images;
- playing simple games such as peek-a-boo;
- use of soft toys and puppets;
- playing of musical instruments;
- use of sensory play including water and textures;
- music therapy, which can also be appropriate for sick or premature neonates.

 Stop and think

Do not forget that siblings can be involved and can be vital to ensure that successful attachment and bonding take place for the whole family. It can be helpful to give siblings a small, achievable task to do for the infant, for example, finding a nappy or infant wipes – they then feel a part of the process. When the infant is older, 'tummy time' with a sibling works well – a sibling can choose a book or a toy to look at with the infant while they (the infant) are lying prone. This is usually a brief period which means that the interaction can be positive, include praise and not last too long.

ATTACHMENT

Attachment is the connection and emotional bond between the infant and their parents. Secure attachment can foster emotional and psychological stability into adulthood and can contribute to the formation of healthy future relationships. Attachment develops over time, starting during the antenatal period, so it is important that early bonding is encouraged during pregnancy. One aspect of attachment is that parents recognise and respond appropriately to their infants' needs by providing timely, appropriate care. This care is loving, responsive and consistent, providing a safe base for infants and children to return to as they explore and develop (Winston and Chicot, 2016). Table 6.3 provides examples of what secure attachment looks like. The effects of insecure attachment may not be evident until childhood or even adulthood; Table 6.4 gives examples of these. Table 6.5 demonstrates what effective bonding and attachment can lead to.

 Table 6.3 Signs of secure attachment

- **Proximity maintenance** – the infant will want to be near their primary caregiver.

- **Safe haven** – the infant will return to their primary caregiver for comfort if they feel frightened or upset.

- **Secure base** – the infant will treat their primary caregiver as a base to explore from, remaining in close proximity so that they can return to that base when needed.

- **Separation anxiety** – the infant will become anxious and distressed in the absence of their primary caregiver and will become upset when they leave.

Adapted from Ainsworth et al (2015)

 Table 6.4 The impact and effects of insecure attachment

Infants and children who have had attachment issues are more likely to:

- develop behavioural problems, which may include attention deficit hyperactivity disorder (ADHD) (Fearon et al, 2010);

- experience difficulty developing healthy friendships and relationships;

- enter into volatile relationships as an adult;

- experience poor mental health in adulthood.

Table 6.5 Effective bonding and attachment

Effective bonding and attachment can lead to:

- improved physical and emotional health for the infant, which facilitates an enhanced skin microbiome, as well as a reduction in illness and cortisol levels (Modak et al, 2023);

- improved emotional health for parents/caregivers;

- improved health outcomes throughout the child's life;

- the formation of healthy future relationships with friends, family and partners;

- the development of emotional intelligence, social skills and enhanced mental health.

 Stop and think

When undertaking the activities suggested to promote attachment and bonding, it is essential not to overwhelm or overstimulate the infant as this may lead to disengagement by the infant. Short activities can be more appropriate and beneficial.

Infants will initiate eye contact but will look away when overwhelmed. Encourage parents to be in tune with their infant's actions and to think about what they might be trying to say.

Potential barriers to healthy and secure attachment and bonding

The bonding and attachment process with a new infant is not always easy. Parents can feel shocked by the transition to parenthood and feel unconfident about how to bond with and care for their infant. Postnatal mood disorders are common and are a potential barrier to bonding and to the optimal development of newborns – this is because parents may struggle to have emotional availability for their infant.

The lack of a parental support network can also have an impact, potentially leading to increased stress and a lack of confidence building as a result of reduced (or absent) peer friendships and support. It is important to offer support and guidance in the antenatal period as elevated stress during this time can hinder the transition into parenthood and impact on the bonding process. Prematurity, or any other complications that cause separation at birth, can also have an impact; in these cases, alternative strategies may be needed and can include the use of bonding squares (small pieces of soft material).

 Refer to Chapter 12 for further information on family care specific to the neonatal unit.

It is important to talk to parents in the early days of parenting. For example, ask them how they are feeling, and facilitate discussions around what their infant is doing, how they are changing and how much comfort they gain from having their parent close. Encouragement is key to supporting bonding and early attachment in line with their cultural preferences. Try to help empower parents on their parenting journey and support them if they are struggling. Table 6.6 identifies some strategies that professionals can use to support families and overcome barriers to bonding and attachment.

 Table 6.6 Strategies that professionals can use to overcome barriers

- Maximise skin-to-skin care in hospital.
- Encourage engagement with parent and infant groups.
- Discuss parental anxieties.
- Facilitate access to appropriate books to read to the infant.
- Role model appropriate communication and behavioural strategies.
- Provide support and education to recognise the infant's cues.
- While cultural and ethnicity should be embraced and not seen as a barrier, always consider if there are any language barriers for non-English speaking families and make arrangements (eg interpretation and translation tools) to ensure understanding and clarity for all parents, whatever their background.

 There are several professionals that can support the family with attachment and bonding; it is important that early identification of individual needs is carried out and relevant referrals made. You can read more about community-based family care in Chapter 15.

 See the web companion for a glossary specific to this chapter.

📍 *Check local variations and guidance alert*

The space below can be used to record any notes or local variations and practice points specific to your own unit.

REFERENCES

Ainsworth, M D, Blehar, M C, Waters, E and Wall, S N (2015) *Patterns of Attachment: A Psychological Study of the Strange Situation*. New York: Psychology Press.

Brown, M, Westerveld, M and Gillon, G (2017) Early Storybook Reading with Infants and Young Children: Parents' Opinions and Home Reading Practices. *Australasian Journal of Early Childhood*, 42(2): 69–77.

Care Quality Commission (CQC) (2022) Culturally Appropriate Care. [online] Available at: www.cqc.org.uk/guidance-providers/adult-social-care/culturally-appropriate-care (accessed 28 January 2024).

Fearon, R P, Bakermans-Kranenburg, M J, Van Ijzendoorn, M H, Lapsley, A and Roisman, G (2010) The Significance of Insecure Attachment and Disorganization in the Development of Children's Externalizing Behavior: A Meta-analytic Study. *Child Development*, 8(2): 435–56.

Harding, C, Whiting, L, Petty, J, Edney, S, Murphy, R and Crossley, S L (2022) Infant Communication: How Should We Define This, and is it Important? *Journal of Neonatal Nursing*, 28(6): 452–4.

International Association of Infant Massage (2023) About Infant Massage. [online] Available at: www.iaim.org.uk/about-infant-massage (accessed 23 January 2024).

Ionio, C, Ciuffo, G and Landoni, M (2021) Parent-Infant Skin-to-Skin Contact and Stress Regulation: A Systematic Review of the Literature. *International Journal of Environmental Research and Public Health*, 18: 1–14.

Modak, A, Ronghe, V and Gomase, K P (2023) The Psychological Benefits of Breastfeeding: Fostering Maternal Well-being and Child Development. *Cureus*, 15(10). [online] Available at: www.cureus.com/articles/187248-the-psychological-benefits-of-breastfeeding-fostering-maternal-well-being-and-child-development#!/ (accessed 19 January 2024).

Moore, E R, Bergman, N, Anderson, G C and Medley, N (2016) Early Skin-to-Skin Contact for Mothers and Their Healthy Newborn Infants (Review). *Cochrane Database of Systematic Reviews*, 11.

Olsson, E, Eriksson, M and Anderzén-Carlsson, A (2017) Skin-to-Skin Contact Facilitates More Equal Parenthood – A Qualitative Study from Fathers' Perspective. *Journal of Pediatric Nursing*, 34: 2–9.

Persico, G, Antolini, L, Vergani, P, Constantini, W, Nardi, M T and Bellotti, L (2017) Maternal Singing of Lullabies During Pregnancy and After Birth: Effects on Mother–Infant Bonding and on Newborns' Behaviour. Concurrent Cohort Study. *Women and Birth*, 30: 214–20.

Vicente, S and Pereira, Â (2021) Infant Massage Programs for Newborn Infants: Systematic Review. *Annals of Medicine (Helsinki)*, 53(1): S145–S146.

Winston, R and Chicot, R (2016) The Importance of Early Bonding on the Long-Term Mental Health and Resilience of Children. *London Journal of Primary Care*, 8(1): 12–14.

Part 2

Caring for the neonate in the clinical setting

Section editor: Julia Petty

7 Altered anatomy and physiology of the neonate

Kathleen Mangahis, Emmie Hopkinson and Julia Petty

INTRODUCTION

The birth of a neonate initiates the transition period between intrauterine to extra-uterine life. This can be a complex process involving major organ and metabolic changes such as the change from foetal to newborn circulation and alteration to the haemodynamics of the cardiovascular system as well as the hepatic, renal and endocrine functions (see Chapter 1). The neonate must assume the role of the 'producer' from being a 'consumer' and take on the functions of the placenta in terms of oxygen transport through the establishment of breathing as well as maintaining glucose and thermal homeostasis. Gestation and other external factors such as the mode of delivery, use of analgesics or anaesthetics, timing of cord clamping, and availability of oxygen, glucose and warmth can have an impact on this process of transition. The successful adaptation from foetal to neonatal life has a large influence on well-being at birth. Any problems encountered at birth or even as late as 24–48 hours post birth due to failure of normal adaptive processes (Hillman et al, 2012; Michel and Lowe, 2017) may lead to problems that require hospital admission. This chapter provides an insight into what happens when normal adaptation at birth is compromised (Figure 7.1) and common conditions presenting in a neonatal unit using a multisystem approach (Table 7.1). Prematurity and respiratory distress syndrome are two commonly seen situations, the focus of Table 7.2 and Figure 7.2, respectively, as examples of specific pathophysiology and related care.

Chapter learning objectives

By the end of this chapter you will:

✓ have an insight into the range of conditions that require admission to a neonatal unit and the associated pathophysiology (altered anatomy and physiology);

✓ be able to consider how altered anatomy and physiology can affect the care of the neonate admitted to hospital.

Critical thinking points

- What are the most common neonatal conditions you have encountered in practice and what signs and symptoms did the neonates present with?

- How do you differentiate each of the conditions from each other?

 Refer to Chapter 1 for an overview of the normal transition to extra-uterine life and the anatomy and physiology of the healthy term neonate.

 See the web companion for supplementary information on delayed and/or compromised transition at birth and associated altered physiology.

COMPROMISE AT BIRTH: THE THREE Hs (HYPOXIA, HYPOTHERMIA, HYPOGLYCAEMIA)

As seen in Chapter 1, at birth, the neonate undergoes transition from the in-utero to ex-utero environment and this depends on the availability of adequate oxygen, energy in the form of glucose and adequate thermal control (Figure 1.1). However, when compromise ensues in the perinatal period, one, two or all three of these elements may be deficient, leading to the potential for hypoxia, hypoglycaemia and/or hypothermia (Morton and Brodsky, 2016; O'Brien and Walker, 2014). Moreover, each element influences the other, as depicted in Figure 7.1.

Stop and think

Prevention of any part of the three Hs triangle is key, achieved through simple, basic care measures (eg early nutrition, avoidance of heat loss and maintaining adequate oxygenation). Any deficiency in any of these three areas will impact negatively on the other two.

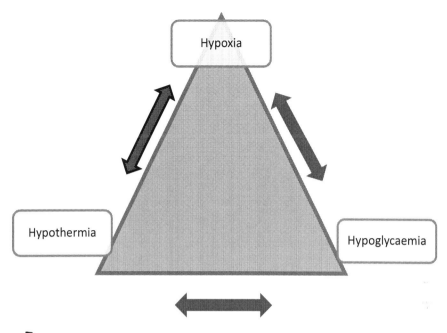

Figure 7.1 The relationship between the 3 Hs: compromise at birth

- ○ **Hypothermia** causes an increase in glucose use, which can lead to hypoglycaemia and increased utilisation of oxygen to warm up which can lead to hypoxia.

- ○ **Hypoxia** depletes oxygen for basic functions such as glucose metabolism and thermogenesis, which can lead to hypoglycaemia and hypothermia.

- ○ **Hypoglycaemia** depletes glucose for basic functions such as respiratory function and thermal control, which can lead to hypoxia and hypothermia.

(Fawcett, 2014; Sharma, 2017)

CONDITIONS THAT MAY BE SEEN IN THE NEONATAL UNIT

There are many conditions that may be seen within a neonatal unit setting, some of which are covered in other chapters. What follows is just a selection of commonly known health issues that require admission and/or further management, relating to altered anatomy and physiology, as compared to the healthy neonate.

Table 7.1 Overview of selected neonatal conditions: altered anatomy and physiology

---

Apnoea: Interruption in breathing, which may be accompanied by bradycardia.

Apnoea of prematurity: A pause of breathing for more than 15–20 s, or accompanied by oxygen desaturation and bradycardia, in infants born before 37 weeks' gestation (Zhao et al, 2011).

Bronchopulmonary dysplasia (BPD): A chronic lung disorder that is most common among premature neonates who received prolonged mechanical ventilation to treat respiratory distress syndrome. BPD is defined as oxygen dependency at 36 weeks corrected age. The term is used synonymously with the term 'chronic lung disease' (National Institute for Health and Care Excellence (NICE), 2019).

Chronic lung disease (CLD): Lung damage and scarring that may occur in neonates treated with oxygen and positive pressure mechanical ventilation for a prolonged period.

Congenital respiratory infection: Due to the immaturity of the immune system, newborn infants, especially preterm babies, are at risk of developing respiratory infections such as pneumonia. These could be acquired through the ascending route associated with prolonged rupture of membranes (PROM), aspiration of vaginal bacteria and the transplacental route. They can present as early or late onset.

Gastro-oesophageal reflux (GOR): Occurs when stomach contents backflow into the oesophagus, leading to irritation and discomfort. It is often caused by under-development of the neuromuscular control of the gastro-oesophageal sphincter.

Intraventricular haemorrhage (IVH): Bleeding in and around the brain's ventricles.

Meconium aspiration syndrome (MAS): Results from the passage of meconium into the amniotic fluid before birth. This will cause the foetus to inhale the meconium, which can lead to the blockage of airways, inflammation within the lungs and decreased oxygenation of the blood, with the neonate showing signs of respiratory distress.

Necrotising enterocolitis (NEC): An acquired, ischaemic, inflammatory condition that causes bowel necrosis, perforation and even death.

Patent ductus arteriosus (PDA): Persistence of the vessel that links the main and left pulmonary arteries and the descending aorta.

Periventricular leukomalacia (PVL): Damage and softening of the white matter within the brain near the cerebral ventricles.

Persistent pulmonary hypertension of the newborn (PPHN): A condition caused by a failure to convert from the foetal circulation pattern to the 'normal' pattern at birth. It occurs when there is a failure to lower the PVR, which leads to continuous right-to-left shunting, hypoxeamia and acidosis.

Pneumonia: A lung infection requiring treatment with antibiotics.

Pneumothorax: The presence of air in the cavity between the lungs and the chest wall (pleural cavity), causing collapse of the lung.

Pulmonary air leak: Any radiologically confirmed air leak serious enough to affect management (including pneumothorax, pulmonary interstitial emphysema, pneumopericardium, pneumoperitoneum and pneumomediastinum).

Pulmonary haemorrhage: Copious bloody secretions in the lung(s) with clinical deterioration requiring change(s) in ventilatory management.

Respiratory distress: Characteristic signs of an inability to breathe effectively including tachypnoea, nasal flaring, grunting, chest recession and an oxygen requirement.

Respiratory distress syndrome (RDS): A condition more commonly seen in premature infants caused by surfactant deficiency and immaturity of the lungs. Without adequate surfactant, the lungs may collapse, which may lead to decreased gas exchange causing signs of respiratory inadequacy.

Respiratory syncytial virus (RSV): RSV commonly causes viral infection in the first year of life, particularly in the winter.

Retinopathy of prematurity (ROP): Blood vessels grow abnormally in the retina, the light-sensitive nerve tissue that lines the inside back wall of the eye.

Transient tachypnoea of the newborn (TTN): A condition where there is a delay in the clearance or reabsorption of foetal lung fluid; it presents at birth and may subside within 24–48 hours, rarely lasting over three to seven days.

(Adapted from various chapters in Boxwell et al, 2020 and El-Radhi, 2015; Gallacher et al, 2016)

 See the web companion for a more detailed table of neonatal conditions with associated assessment, diagnosis and management.

For care guidance, refer to the following guidelines: NICE (2019) 'Specialist neonatal respiratory care for babies born preterm' and Sweet et al (2023) 'European consensus guidelines on the management of respiratory distress syndrome', as well as your own individual unit guidelines.

THE PRETERM INFANT: ALTERED ANATOMY AND PHYSIOLOGY

The preterm infant is compared to the term neonate below, according to the same systems highlighted in Table 1.2, Chapter 1.

⊞ Table 7.2 Overview of the systems: altered physiology of the preterm neonate

System	Preterm neonate
Respiratory	• Undeveloped respiratory centre, resulting in a predisposition to apnoea.
	• Immature pulmonary function from less alveoli growth means reduced surface area for gaseous exchange and lower lung functional residual capacity.
	• Alveoli are more fragile with high surface tension.
	• Risk of surfactant deficiency.
	• Increased risk to damaged lungs from mechanical ventilation.
Cardiovascular and haematological	• Total blood volume is reduced.
	• Red blood cells have a shorter life span of approx. 30–40 days.
	• There is a more rapid decline in haemoglobin.
	• Clotting times are extended.
	• Greater risk of reduction of cardiac contractility.
	• Less sensitivity to constricting effects of oxygen at birth to close the ductus arteriosus, which may lead to this space remaining open.
Immune	• Prematurity causes a higher risk of immature specific and non-specific immune systems.
Digestive	• The digestive tract is less mature in relation to intestine length, absorptive ability and motility.
	• The risk of gastro-oesophageal reflux is greater in preterm neonates.
Hepatic	• The lower the gestation, the greater risk of slowed liver metabolism.
	• Greater risk of physiological jaundice due to liver enzyme immaturity and lower treatment thresholds.
	• Reduced clotting factors and ability to metabolise drugs and other agents.

System	Preterm neonate
Fluid balance/ renal and urinary-genital	• The kidneys are immature in relation to tubule function with more limited ability than term neonates to filtrate large volumes and predisposition to fluid overload is more common. • Sodium loss is common in the preterm neonate due to limited ability to conserve this via the kidneys. • Differences may be seen in the genitalia due to immaturity – eg the testes may not have descended and the labia majora may not cover the minora, depending on gestational age.
Thermoregulatory	• At early gestation (less than 30 weeks), they lack adipose tissue (brown fat), which is a necessary component for heat generation through non-shivering thermogenesis, and are therefore at a greater risk of poor thermoregulation. • Skin lacks keratin (waterproofing layer) with a greater risk of evaporative heat and water loss. • They will also be lacking in subcutaneous tissue, which is insulation underneath the skin that assists in preventing heat loss. • There is a reduced ability to adapt to the extra-uterine environment after birth, which can lead to a greater risk of hypothermia.
Metabolism	• There are much more limited glycogen stores in a preterm that may also lack nutritional reserves (fat, iron and vitamins) which are usually introduced in the third trimester of pregnancy. • There is a greater inability to achieve normal metabolic adaptation to extra-uterine life due to developmental immaturity.
Neurological	• There is a greater risk of neurological injury due to an immature germinal matrix within the ventricles before 34 weeks' gestation and an immature vascular cerebral blood supply. Therefore, there is a greater risk to bleeding and ischaemic damage to the brain. • There is an increased inability for autoregulation in response to compromise such as maintaining adequate cerebral perfusion in the event of low systemic blood pressure. • The preterm neonate has an underdeveloped brain stem along with an increased sensitivity of the vagus nerve. This leads to an increased risk of apnoea, bradycardia and immature chemoreceptor responses to hypoxia and increased CO_2.

→

Table 7.2 (cont.)

System	Preterm neonate
Sensory	• Sensory, pain and behavioural systems are immature and behaviours may not follow the usual expected patterns as seen in term neonates. • Sensory function is at greater risk of damage as this is still developing, eg the vascular layer of the retina, visual and auditory nerves are prone to damage from various risk factors.
Behavioural	• The sensory, pain and behavioural systems are immature, which may lead to behaviours that do not follow the usual expected patterns seen in the neonatal period.
Musculoskeletal	• A preterm neonate born before 34 weeks' gestation has reduced tone, lacking physiological flexion, and shows an extended posture with limbs lying straight and flat.
Integumentary	• Lack of collagen in the skin leads to the skin being fragile, transparent and easily damaged. • Very preterm neonates will exhibit signs of immature gestation such as flat nipples, reduced/absent palmar and plantar creases, a lack of cartilage in the soft pinna of the ear and visible lanugo hair at around 24–28 weeks' gestation up to 32 weeks before diminishing.

(Kilby et al, 2020)

An example of altered neonatal anatomy and physiology: respiratory distress

The term 'respiratory distress' describes a set of symptoms related to breathing problems and can present with a variety of conditions. 'Respiratory distress syndrome' is a diagnosis defined as a lack of endogenous surfactant and is a prevalent condition in the neonatal unit particularly among the preterm population, with specific management (Figure 7.2).

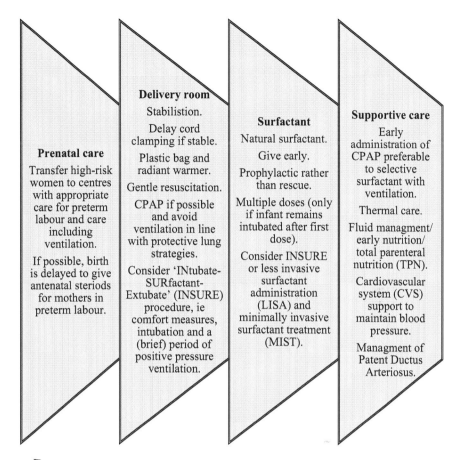

Prenatal care

Transfer high-risk women to centres with appropriate care for preterm labour and care including ventilation.

If possible, birth is delayed to give antenatal steriods for mothers in preterm labour.

Delivery room

Stabilistion.

Delay cord clamping if stable.

Plastic bag and radiant warmer.

Gentle resuscitation.

CPAP if possible and avoid ventilation in line with protective lung strategies.

Consider 'INtubate-SURfactant-Extubate' (INSURE) procedure, ie comfort measures, intubation and a (brief) period of positive pressure ventilation.

Surfactant

Natural surfactant.

Give early.

Prophylactic rather than rescue.

Multiple doses (only if infant remains intubated after first dose).

Consider INSURE or less invasive surfactant administration (LISA) and minimally invasive surfactant treatment (MIST).

Supportive care

Early administration of CPAP preferable to selective surfactant with ventilation.

Thermal care.

Fluid managment/ early nutrition/ total parenteral nutrition (TPN).

Cardiovascular system (CVS) support to maintain blood pressure.

Managment of Patent Ductus Arteriosus.

 Figure 7.2 Overview of care principles for respiratory distress syndrome (RDS). Signs of 'respiratory distress'/RDS: tachypnoea, nasal flaring, intercostal recession, apnoea, cyanosis/pallor, poor oxygen saturations, oxygen requirement and grunting. Remember to consider the skin tone and ethnicity of the neonate when assessing for cyanosis as this is more difficult to identify in darker skins (see Chapters 4 and 10)

(NICE, 2019; Sweet et al, 2023)

📍 *Check local guidance*

Ensure you check your individual guidelines as there may be some variations in practice in terms of management of RDS, surfactant administration and other conditions in this chapter.

The following aspects should be considered during surfactant administration.

○ Preparation of surfactant – natural preparation is kept in the refrigerator and requires warming before use. It should not be shaken.

○ Use minimal or non-invasive means of administration where possible – eg LISA/MIST (Herting et al, 2019).

○ If surfactant is administered down the endotracheal tube, ideally the position should be confirmed beforehand to avoid an erroneous instillation into one lung.

○ Perform endotracheal tube (ETT) suction prior to administration *only if required* and avoid afterwards.

○ It is important to watch for bradycardia or desaturation during administration.

○ Neonates on high-frequency ventilation may be given surfactant without disconnection if suitable T-piece connectors are available.

○ Following administration, lung compliance may improve quite quickly, and ventilator requirements need to be monitored and weaned to prevent overinflation.

○ Repeat dosing – following the administration of the initial dose of surfactant, the timing and necessity for further doses should be decided on an individual basis.

Non-standard use: Surfactant might be used in other conditions including meconium aspiration syndrome, congenital pneumonia, pulmonary haemorrhage (Sweet et al, 2023) or PPHN to improve oxygenation. This decision is decided on a case-by-case basis.

 Stop and think

The importance of non-invasive means of respiratory support (INSURE, LISA, MIST) is emphasised whatever the cause of respiratory distress – ie to protect the lungs and prevent long-term damage (Sweet et al, 2023). When giving surfactant, watch closely for changes to oxygenation and chest expansion.

Standard precautions alert

Prevention is still the best intervention when caring for infants in the neonatal unit; for example, the utilisation of infection control practices and aseptic non-touch technique will help prevent the spread of infection. Remember that early detection is important to ensure appropriate interventions are put into place.

 See the web companion for a glossary specific to this chapter.

 ## Check local variations and guidance alert

The space below can be used to record any notes or local variations and practice points specific to your own unit.

REFERENCES

Boxwell, G, Petty, J and Kaiser, L (eds) (2020) *Neonatal Intensive Care Nursing*. 3rd edn. New York: Routledge.

El-Radhi, A S (2015) Management of Common Neonatal Problems. *British Journal of Nursing*, 24(5): 258–5.

Fawcett, K (2014) Preventing Admission Hypothermia in Very Low Birth Weight Neonates. *Neonatal Network*, 33(3): 143–9.

Gallacher, D J, Hart, K and Kotecha, S (2016) Common Respiratory Conditions of the Newborn. *Breathe*, 12: 30–42.

Herting, E, Härtel, C and Göpel, W (2019) Less Invasive Surfactant Administration (LISA): Chances and Limitations. *Archives of Disease in Childhood – Fetal and Neonatal Edition*, 104: F655–F659.

Hillman, N H, Kallapur, S G and Jobe, A H (2012) Physiology of Transition from Intrauterine to Extrauterine Life. *Clinics in Perinatology*, 39(4): 769–83.

Kilby, L, Everett, E, Powis, K and Kyte, E (2020) The Preterm and Low Birthweight Infant. In Boxwell, G, Petty, J and Kaiser, L (eds) *Neonatal Intensive Care Nursing*. 3rd ed (Chapter 3). Abingdon: Routledge.

Michel, A and Lowe, N K (2017) The Successful Immediate Neonatal Transition to Extrauterine Life. *Biological Research for Nursing*, 19(3): 287–94.

Morton, S U and Brodsky, D (2016) Fetal Physiology and the Transition to Extrauterine Life. *Clinics in Perinatology*, 43(3): 395–407.

National Institute for Health and Care Excellence (NICE) (2019) Specialist Neonatal Respiratory Care for Babies Born Preterm: NICE Guideline [NG124]. [online] Available at: www.nice.org.uk/guidance/ng124 (accessed 1 November 2023).

O'Brien, F and Walker, I A (2014) Fluid Homeostasis in the Neonate. *Pediatric Anesthesia*, 24(1): 49–59.

Sharma, D (2017) Golden Hour of Neonatal Life: Need of the Hour. *Maternal Health, Neonatology, and Perinatology*, 3: 16.

Sweet, D G, Carnielli, V P, Greisen, G et al (2023) European Consensus Guidelines on the Management of Respiratory Distress Syndrome: 2022 Update. *Neonatology*, 120(1): 3–23.

Zhao, J, Gonzalez, F and Mu, D (2011) Apnea of Prematurity: From Cause to Treatment. *European Journal of Pediatrics*, 170(9): 1097–105.

8 Important principles of care in the neonatal unit

Michelle Scott, Melanie Carpenter and Julia Petty

INTRODUCTION

When a newborn is born prematurely or unwell, requiring admission to a neonatal unit, there are various fundamental areas of care to address whatever dependency level they are admitted to and nursed within, be it intensive, high-dependency or special care. This chapter covers important principles of care that are relevant to all dependency levels within the neonatal unit setting specifically, namely, thermal care, blood sugar monitoring, oxygen therapy, fluid balance, feeding and nutrition, skin and wound care, infection control and care of the jaundiced neonate (Figures 8.1 to 8.12; Tables 8.1 to 8.18).

Chapter learning objectives

By the end of this chapter you will:

✓ have gained insight into key areas of essential practice relevant to all dependency levels on the neonatal unit;

✓ understand essential practice points required for infants in the neonatal unit, in relation to thermoregulation, blood glucose monitoring, oxygen therapy, fluid balance and feeding, skin care, infection and jaundice using an inclusive approach to care.

Critical thinking points

- Related to the altered physiology discussed in Chapter 7, consider how this impacts on the care delivered to a neonate admitted to the neonatal unit.

- Consider the above areas of care in relation to the different dependency levels through the whole neonatal unit journey.

For practices relating to the well neonate, please refer to Chapters 2 and 5 (eg skin care, infection prevention, feeding and jaundice).

 See the web companion for supplementary information on the topics covered throughout this chapter.

NEONATAL THERMAL CARE

As soon as a baby is born, they are exposed to a significantly cooler extra-uterine environment and so thermal care is a vital consideration. All neo-nates/infants, due to their physiological immaturity, are predisposed to heat loss and vulnerability is even greater in the premature neonate (Turnbull and Petty, 2013). Neonatal hypothermia has been associated with increased risk of mortality and morbidity, which can be avoided by simple, fundamental measures to limit heat loss (Lyu et al, 2015; McCall et al, 2018); therefore, thermal care following delivery is essential, summarised in Figures 8.1 to 8.4 and Tables 8.1 to 8.2.

 Stop and think

A neonate's core temperature should be always maintained between 36.5 and 37.5 degrees Celsius (°C) (Sweet et al, 2023). The rec-ommendation for the minimum central temperature on admission to the neonatal unit from the labour ward or other, is 36°C (British Association of Perinatal Medicine (BAPM), 2019).

Table 8.1 Heat loss methods and related thermal care

Sources of heat loss	Example	Preventative measures
CONDUCTION **Direct transfer of heat from the neonate to a cooler object.**	Contact with a cold surface, such as scales or stethoscope.	Use of warmed blankets/towels, ie cover scales with a warm blanket/ towel.
		Hat.

Sources of heat loss	Example	Preventative measures
		Heated mattress, radiant warmer.
		Warmed intravenous therapy solutions, gases and stethoscopes.
CONVECTION **The loss of heat from an object to the surrounding air of a cool environment; air movement across the neonate's skin surface.**	Draughts or cooler environment; use of non-humidified oxygen.	Room temperature for delivery should be 26°C (BAPM, 2019), neonatal unit 20–26°C and after discharge home, 18°C.
		Place neonate within a pre-warmed incubator (Figure 8.1).
		Keep infant covered and avoid draughts near doorways and windows.
RADIATION **Heat radiating towards a cooler surface not in direct contact.**	Cold incubator doors.	Prewarm incubator.
		Keep neonate away from cold surfaces or objects.
		Radiant heater during stabilisation/procedures.
EVAPORATION **Moisture from body surfaces – a liquid-to-air vapour**	Following delivery, amniotic fluid; after a bath.	Plastic bags/wrap (<28–30 weeks and/or <1 kg (Figure 8.2)).
		Dry and wrap >30 weeks neonate at birth.
		Humification within incubators.
		Change wet clothing linen, ie following vomiting, washing.
ALL	Ensure a neutral thermal environment (NTE) is set within the incubator (Table 8.2 and Figure 8.3) and maintained at all dependency levels (Figure 8.4); in addition, 'Servo' or manual control can be used for incubator temperatures.	

(Turnbull and Petty, 2013; McCall et al, 2018; Wood et al, 2022)

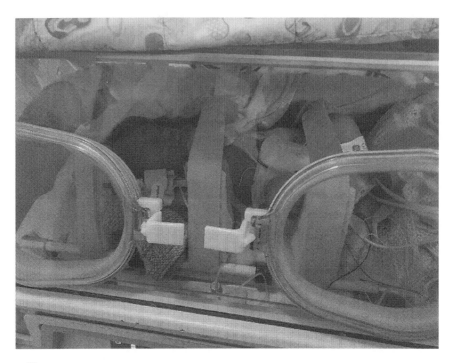

↗ Figure 8.1 Premature neonate in an incubator

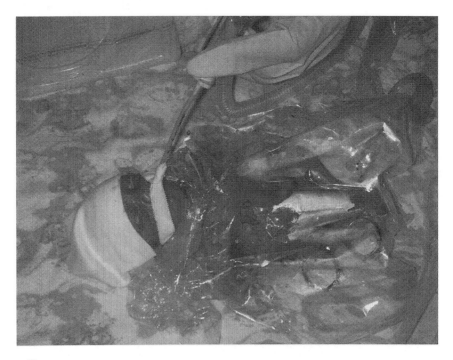

↗ Figure 8.2 Premature infant placed into a plastic bag
(Reproduced with the kind permission of Resuscitation Council UK)

Stop and think

Incubator care (double walled – Figure 8.3) is the optimum method of providing a neutral thermal environment (NTE) in the first instance at a time when thermal control is limited. Age and gestation must be considered to set the desired incubator (environmental) temperature with minimal oxygen and energy consumption by the neonate (Gardner et al, 2020).

⊞ Table 8.2 Neutral thermal environment guide

Age	1000–1200 grams (+ or – 0.5°C)	1200–1500 grams (+ or – 0.5°C)	1500–2500 grams (+ or – 1.0°C)	>2500 & >36 wks. (+ or – 1.5°C)
0–12 hrs	35	34	33.3	32.8
12–24 hrs	34.5	33.8	32.8	32.4
24–96 hrs	34.5	33.5	32.3	32

Age	<1500 grams (+ or – 1.5°C)	1500–2500 grams (+ or – 1.5°C)	>2500 & >36 weeks (+ or – 1.5°C)
5–14 days	33.5	32.1	32
2–3 wks	33.1	31.7	30
3–4 wks	32.6	31.4	<30
4–5 wks	32	30.9	<30
5–6 wks	31.4	30.4	<30

(Gardner et al, 2020)

(NB + or – relates to the range: ie + or – 0.5°C means plus or minus 0.5°C)

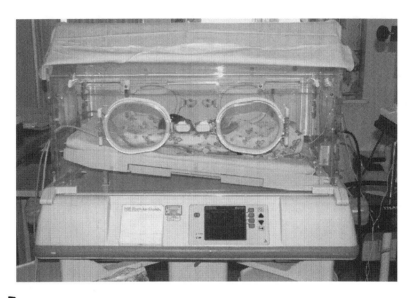

Figure 8.3 Double-walled incubator

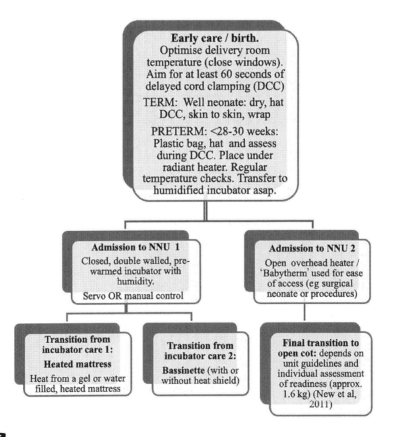

Early care / birth.
Optimise delivery room temperature (close windows). Aim for at least 60 seconds of delayed cord clamping (DCC)

TERM: Well neonate: dry, hat DCC, skin to skin, wrap

PRETERM: <28-30 weeks: Plastic bag, hat and assess during DCC. Place under radiant heater. Regular temperature checks. Transfer to humidified incubator asap.

Admission to NNU 1
Closed, double walled, pre-warmed incubator with humidity.
Servo OR manual control

Admission to NNU 2
Open overhead heater / 'Babytherm' used for ease of access (eg surgical neonate or procedures)

Transition from incubator care 1:
Heated mattress
Heat from a gel or water filled, heated mattress

Transition from incubator care 2:
Bassinette (with or without heat shield)

Final transition to open cot: depends on unit guidelines and individual assessment of readiness (approx. 1.6 kg) (New et al, 2011)

Figure 8.4 Methods of keeping neonates warm through the dependency levels

Check local guidance

Observe local guidance on humidification procedure.

 Stop and think

Generally, a neonate <26–30 weeks, <1 kg in weight, in the first 7–10 days should be nursed in 60–70 per cent relative humidity via a closed incubator. For <26 weeks' gestation, up to 95 per cent can be given and discontinued once the neonate has developed a skin barrier at approximately two weeks postnatal age (Glass and Valdez, 2021; Sweet et al, 2023).

 Refer to the web companion for more detail on humidification in thermal care.

BLOOD GLUCOSE MONITORING

Blood glucose is the main energy source essential for all bodily functions and its analysis is a common test within neonatal care. A healthy term baby, if kept warm and fed within the first few hours of birth, should be able to control their own blood glucose. However, during compromise, stress or illness, a neonate may not be able to mount this normal metabolic adaptation when glucose levels drop. Table 8.3 addresses blood glucose monitoring.

 Table 8.3 Blood glucose monitoring in the neonatal unit

HYPOGLYCAEMIA

Identify the 'at-risk' infant.

- Preterm gestation, small for gestational age, low birth weight (<2.5 kg), maternal diabetes, intrapartum asphyxia, resuscitation at birth, sick infants (eg infection), hypothermia.

Ensure ongoing observation and documented monitoring.

- Signs to observe for: altered level of consciousness, apnoea, cyanosis, hypothermia, jitteriness, convulsions, reduced tone (Cranmer, 2022).

Operational threshold defined as 2.5 mmol/litre (see below).

- This is a consensus based on evidence (BAPM, 2024).

Table 8.3 (cont.)

The feeding infant

- At-risk infants should feed as soon as possible after birth and at frequent intervals until feeding maintains their *pre-feed* blood glucose levels at the desired level. An example would be an infant born to a diabetic mother (IDM).

- Additional measures such as tube feeding (for 'top-ups' with expressed breast milk or formula milk) or intravenous dextrose should be implemented only *if necessary* – eg when abnormal clinical signs occur or if an infant will not orally feed effectively.

The infant with hypoglycaemia in intensive care who is unable to feed.

- Intravenous dextrose (IV) 10% is given firstly as a bolus (2–2.5 ml/kg) followed by maintenance fluids according to the individual infant's condition.

- Higher dextrose concentrations may be required.

- Monitoring of blood glucose (once to twice hourly until stable) and titration of IV glucose.

- Blood glucose below 1.1 mmol/L – refer as an emergency and treat immediately.

HYPERGLYCAEMIA

- Premature infants can be prone to hyperglycaemia due to immature ability to tolerate glucose or as a biochemical sign of stress.

- The most common definition is a blood glucose of >10 mmol/L (Alsweiler et al, 2007; Beardsall, 2021).

- A common consensus in the evidence is that over 8 mmol/L should be avoided (Beardsall, 2021).

- The decision whether to treat or not with insulin, however, is determined by both blood glucose and accompanying glycosuria (>1%).

 Stop and think

The operational threshold in the treatment of hypoglycaemia; in the high-risk infant, is:

- a value <1.0 mmol/L at any time;

- a single value <2.5 mmol/L in an infant with abnormal clinical signs;

- a value <2.0 mmol/L and remaining <2.0 mmol/L at the next measurement in an infant with a risk factor for impaired metabolic adaptation and hypoglycaemia but without abnormal clinical signs (BAPM, 2024).

Check local guidance

Check local guidance on acceptable glucose norms and blood glucose monitoring procedures.

OXYGEN THERAPY

The goal of oxygen therapy is to achieve adequate delivery of oxygen to the tissue without creating oxygen toxicity. A failure to maintain adequate blood oxygen levels can result in progressive deterioration. Figures 8.5 to 8.6 and Tables 8.4 to 8.5 focus on methods of oxygen administration, oxygen monitoring and understanding parameters/limits. The administration of oxygen to infants requires the selection of an oxygen delivery system that suits the weight, age and the clinical need.

Facial	Ambient
For short term administration only; for example, during resuscitation at birth when required administered with BVM or t-piece. With BVM, quantity delivered not known. With t-piece, use air/oxygen blender Always start reuscitation in air and give oxygen according to saturation readlings.	Into incubator for up to 30% oxygen requirement. The incubator will display the percentage delivered. No need to humidify if<30%. Consider CPAP (depending also on blood gases and other assessment criteria). Remember to check the percentage delivered with an oxygen analyser which should be calibrated to zero prior to use.

Neonatal oxygen therapy

High flow nasal cannula oxygen	Low-flow nasal cannula oxygen
Delivery of blended oxygen and air at flow rates of > 1 L/min (1-8) (Wilkinson et al, 2011), for example, via the Vapotherm© device, a thermally controlled humidification system (at 95% or greater relative humidity) that flushes nasopharyngeal dead space. Temperature setting must be 37°C when flow rates >4 LPM and 34–35°C with flow rates <4 LPM. Change water.	For low-flow oxygen <1 litre/minute. The cannula is connected to a wall oxygen connection via a flow meter. Can be humidified if necessary (depending on flow). Read from the centre of the ball in the flow meter; document and record volume being delivered. Necessary for home oxygen therapy.

 Figure 8.5 Neonatal oxygen therapy

⊞ Table 8.4 Overview of oxygen monitoring methods

Method	How does it work?	Considerations
Arterial blood	Measures actual tissue oxygen as a partial pressure (kPa or mmHg) via invasive means through aspiration of blood from an in-dwelling arterial line for blood gas analysis.	Invasive.
Oxygen saturation (SpO_2) via pulse oximetry **(Figure 8.6)**	Measures the absorption of red and infrared light by pulsatile blood. The relative absorption of light by oxyhaemoglobin and deoxyhaemoglobin is processed by the device and an oxygen saturation level is reported. The result is a continuous qualitative measurement of oxyhaemoglobin (%).	Change probe site regularly (at least four times hourly). Ensure pulsatile trace.
Transcutaneous oxygen ($TcPO_2$)	A heated probe applied to the skin measures the 'arterialised' partial pressure values (through the skin) of the underlying capillaries reflecting tissue oxygenation in kPa. This method can also monitor transcutaneous CO_2.	Calibration is required at each site change (two to four times hourly).
Pre and post ductal PaO_2 or SpO_2 monitoring	Pulse oximetry or blood gas analysis from the upper (pre-ductal via right hand) and lower/umbilical (post-ductal) body can help identify a right-to-left shunt occurring through the ductus arteriosus.	Typically, a difference in upper limb pre- and post-ductal measurements suggests a right-to-left shunt.
Oxygenation index (OI)	A calculated value to determine an infant's oxygen demand and associated level of oxygenation. $$OI= \frac{MAP\ (cm\ H_2O) \times FiO_2 \times 100}{PaO_2\ (mmHg)}$$	Used as criteria for nitric oxide or more advanced interventions in the very sick newborn.

 Stop and think

Term infants who require resuscitation should be given air and then oxygen delivered *according to need* and O_2 saturations, before being weaned as soon as possible. Remember that oxygen is a drug with potential risks. An infant receiving oxygen via any means should be monitored by pulse oximetry to assess the efficacy of the therapy and to guide the dose.

Check local guidance

Check local guidance and policy on oxygen monitoring and setting alarm limits.

 Stop and think

Monitoring of both oxygen delivery and the levels in the blood and tissues is essential to guard against the risk of too little or too much oxygen, both of which have related physiological effects.

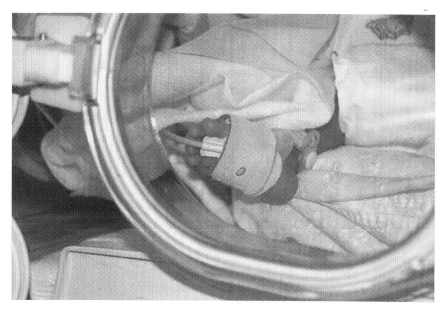

 Figure 8.6 Oxygen saturation probe

 Stop and think

Setting appropriate upper and lower limits for oxygen monitoring should be done in line with age, gestation and whether oxygen or air is being required – for example, one can be more liberal with the set limits if an infant is no longer at risk of retinopathy of prematurity (ROP) and/or once he/she is in air (Cherian et al, 2014).

Table 8.5 Setting oxygen targets

Arterial blood – taken from blood gas analysis. 6.5–10 kPa (neonatal).

Transcutaneous – as for blood gas. 6.5–10 kPa (preterm)/6.5–12 kPa (term).

Oxygen saturations

- After 10 minutes of life, for a saturation target of 90 to 94%, set lower and upper alarm limits at 89% and 95% respectively (Sweet et al, 2023) (subject to local variations) for premature infants requiring oxygen before their eyes have vascularised fully.

- For premature infants in air or out of ROP risk, the upper limit can be set higher.

- Keep limits 95–100% in term infants and those that have pulmonary hypertension.

(Sweet et al, 2023)

*NB UK Resuscitation Council (2021) guidance for pre-ductal saturations in the first 10 minutes of life: 2 minutes 65%, 5 minutes 85%, 10 minutes 90%

FLUID BALANCE

Optimum fluid management is about ensuring a balance between input and output. Neonatal fluid management will change and adapt based on age, weight, maintenance needs, deficits and ongoing losses. It is a vital part of neonatal care and is not always straightforward in a sick and/or premature infant (Moss, 2022). Guidance around calculating fluids, electrolytes and daily allowances is summarised in Table 8.6. Table 8.7 provides an overview of how we monitor renal function, which includes an understanding of urinalysis.

 Table 8.6 Calculating fluids and daily allowances

- Calculate fluids on birth weight (BW) until it is regained, and then base the calculation on *current* weight. Expect up to 10 per cent weight loss from BW in term infants and 7–10 per cent in very low birth weight (VLBW) and extremely low birth weight (ELBW) infants, before BW is regained.

- Most infants should be started on intravenous fluids of 70–80 ml/kg/day. Fluids must be tailored individually according to serum sodium levels, urine output and weight loss (Sweet et al, 2023).

- Total volumes of fluid include all infusions and/or enteral feeds, but not usually including bolus drugs or volume.

- A gradual increase of fluid intake is recommended after birth. An example of a basic fluid regime is given below.

- Multiply the required daily volume by weight and divide by 24 hours to obtain hourly input.

	Day 1	Day 2	Day 3	Day 4	Day 5	
Term infant	40–60	50–70	60–80	60–100	100–140	ml/kg/day
Premature infant >1500 g	60–80	80–100	100–120	120–140	140–160	ml/kg/day
Premature infant 1000 g–1500 g	70–90	90–110	110–130	130–150	160–180	ml/kg/day
Premature infant >1000 g	80–100	100–120	120–140	140–160	160–180	ml/kg/day

- Exceptions: hypoglycaemia (higher), birth asphyxia (restricted)
- Weight is an important parameter for fluid requirement assessment.
- After initial weight loss, BW should usually be regained by day 7–10.
- Monitoring: the lower the gestation at birth, the greater the frequency of monitoring required.
- Infants receiving intravenous (IV) fluids and parenteral nutrition (PN) should have weight and serum electrolytes measured at least daily.
- Monitor output: urine output should be a minimum of 1 ml/kg/day on day 1, then 2–3 ml/kg/day thereafter. Weigh nappies (1 g = 1 ml urine).
- Fluid balance along with weight are both important in making decisions about liberalising/increasing fluids.
- Needs of individual infants may deviate from the ranges of recommended fluid intakes depending on clinical circumstances such as fluid retention, dehydration or excessive water losses.

(Jochum et al, 2018)

Intravenous infusion care bundle

✓ Handwashing.

✓ Assess need for IV cannula/central line.

✓ Site inspection hourly and document.

✓ Use visual infusion phlebitis (VIP) score and document.

✓ If lines are not required, remove.

✓ Access – use aseptic non-touch technique (ANTT).

✓ Clean all ports with alcohol swab and allow to dry.

> **See the web companion for information on glucose and electrolyte requirements, giving electrolytes and care of intravenous access sites including VIP scoring.**

Stop and think

Electrolytes should be prescribed and administered according to individual need, evaluated on a regular basis. Care must be taken when administering electrolytes intravenously as they are *hypertonic* solutions, potentially causing significant damage to the tissue if there is any extravasation. Observe the IV site regularly.

⊞ Table 8.7 Renal monitoring and urinalysis

Urine collection methods

Urine bag

Cotton wool balls in nappy

Suprapubic aspiration of bladder (only if necessary)

Catheterisation (rarely)

Ward-based urinalysis

Dipstick urinalysis provides information about multiple physiochemical properties of urine.

pH	The average urine is slightly acidic and usually 5–6 but can vary from 4.8–8.5. Urine pH can be helpful in the diagnosis of renal problems/competency, metabolic disturbances and blood gas compensation.
Specific gravity	A quick and convenient test for monitoring the concentrating and diluting power of the kidney, recognising dehydration and fluid overload. Range = 1.000 to 1.030. Low concentration (nearer 1.000) may be caused by high fluid intake. High concentration (nearer 1.030) may be caused by inadequate fluid intake.
Bilirubin	Presence of bilirubin is indicative of hepatic disease.
Urobilinogen	Normally present in urine at 0.1–1.9 mg/dL.
Protein	Urine can contain a very small amount of protein (trace), but high levels can indicate infection, renal disease and immature kidneys. The result should be negative or show no more than a trace amount of protein.

Blood	Presence of blood suggests renal disease and/or infection or bleeding disorders. The result should be negative.
Ketones	Breakdown products of fatty acid metabolism caused by inadequate nutrition. The result should be negative.
Glucose	Presence of glucose is indicative of hyperglycaemia, stress, metabolic disorders and renal incompetency. The result should be negative.

Other laboratory urine tests

Culture (infection screen), osmolarity (concentration), sodium (abnormal losses from kidneys), metabolites (tests for metabolic disease), toxicology (tests for illicit drug use from maternal transfer to infant).

Signs of renal failure/compromise

Plasma creatinine is the most widely used marker of renal function.

Urine output should be a *minimum* of 0.5–1 ml/kg/hour.

Weight/serum sodium and potassium/blood urea nitrogen.

(Moss, 2022)

 Stop and think

Ward-based urinalysis provides useful information on hydration levels, potential infection and tolerance to glucose. It should not be overlooked when an infant is sick in intensive care and used along with key laboratory testing as necessary.

FEEDING AND NUTRITION IN THE NEONATAL UNIT

A healthy infant will feed responsively via either breast or bottle without difficulty. However, in neonatal care, feeding management and support is necessary for sick and immature infants. Establishing postnatal nutrition is an essential part of neonatal care (Tume et al, 2020), covered in Figures 8.7 to 8.9 and Table 8.8.

Intensive care
- Intravenous (IV) fluids (glucose)
- Total parenteral nutrition (TPN)
- Start enteral nutrition as early as possible
- Trophic feeding (minimal enteral nutrition) is extra to IV volumes using breast milk

High dependency
- Enteral tube (gavage) via nasogastric tube (Figure 8.8) or orogastric tube.
- Bolus (gavage) feeding or continuous in specific situtations (severe reflux)
- Breast milk is preferable to formula if possible
- Other methods of feeding may be required for surgical reasons, eg gastrostomy

Special care
- When ready, start transition to oral feeding (usually around 34 weeks corrected gestation)
- Use non-nutritive sucking with a pacifier in the transition to oral feeding (Figure 8.9)
- The ideal method is breastfeeding with support in line with UNICEF (2016) Baby Friendly Guidelines
- If formula fed, use special formulas and/or supplementation as appropriate for gestation, weight and nutritional status

 Figure 8.7 Overview of feeding methods

 Stop and think

The aim is always to feed an infant *as early as possible* if their physiological condition, gestation and ability to tolerate enteral feeding allows.

 Table 8.8 Nutritional requirements in the infant

An infant requires the following for adequate growth.

Carbohydrate	Protein	Lipids	Vitamins

Lipids: long chain polyunsaturated fatty acids (DHA and AA)

Vitamins: thiamine, riboflavin, niacin, vitamin B12, folate, vitamin C, vitamin A, vitamin D

Minerals: calcium, phosphorus, magnesium, sodium, potassium, chloride, iron, zinc, copper, selenium and iodine

Optimum energy to protein ratio (see below)

Nutrient	Term		Preterm
Energy (kcal/kg/day)	96–120		115–140
Protein (g/kg/day)	2.1		3.5–4.5 <1 kg 4–4.5
Energy:protein ratio		1–1.8 kg	12.8–14.4%
		<1 kg	14.4–16.4%

Type of nutrition

- Parenteral nutrition should be started from birth. Amino acids 1.5–2 g/kg/day should be started from day 1 and built up to 2.5–3.5 g/kg/day (B2). Lipids 1–2 g/kg/day should be started from day 1 and built up to 4.0 g/kg/day as tolerated (Sweet et al, 2023).

- Enteral feeding with mother's milk should be started from the first day if the infant is hemodynamically stable. Breast milk is always the preferred choice of milk.

- If parents choose not to breast feed, education and support should also be given in relation to safe administration of formula milk.

- For premature infants (<34 weeks' gestation), breast milk fortifier can be added at an agreed time once they are able to tolerate 120–150 ml/kg/day.

- If there is insufficient or no expressed breast milk (EBM), preterm formula can be used for infants born less than 34 weeks' gestation. Infants greater than 34 weeks can be given term formula.

- Donor breast milk (DBM) can be used where available, particularly if there is poor tolerance of formula milk or while awaiting maternal EBM supply to increase.

- Older premature infants (>34 weeks) can be breastfed, given EBM or term formula is given if breastfeeding is not chosen or EBM is not available.

(Embleton et al, 2023)

 Check local guidance

All the above decisions are subject to local policy and individualised assessment of weight gain and growth. Check local guidance for agreed procedure for supplementation and choice of feeding/milk.

See the web companion for information on handling/storage of expressed breast milk, making up formula feeds, giving total parenteral nutrition (TPN), trophic feeding, advancement of enteral feeds and insertion/checking naso/orogastric feeding tubes.

 Stop and think

Any specific nutritional advice should be discussed with the neonatal dietician as an important member of the multi-disciplinary team.

Standard precautions alert

Strict infection control should be adhered to in relation to handling of any milk preparation.

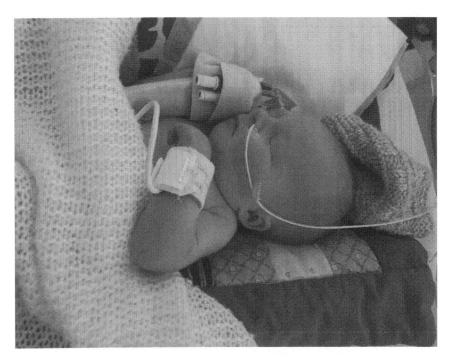

 Figure 8.8 Neonate with nasogastric feeding tube

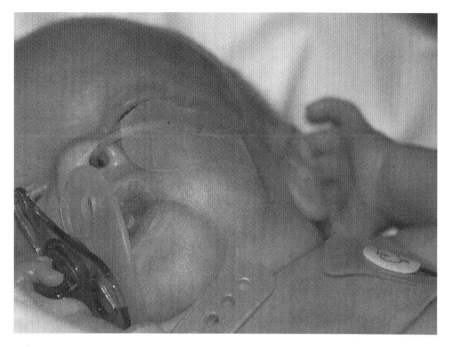

Figure 8.9 Neonate using a pacifier for non-nutritive sucking

SKIN CARE IN THE NEONATAL UNIT

The skin of a newborn, particularly if born preterm, has a relatively poor barrier function with a greater risk of injury from pressure and shearing forces than older infants and children (Oranges et al, 2015). This can increase the risk of infection, discomfort, excoriation or epidermal stripping, particularly if the skin is oedematous because of illness. Skin care assessment can therefore be challenging, particularly in neonates with black or brown skin tones from diverse ethnic backgrounds (Carter et al, 2023) where there is often less understanding and limited guidance (Carter et al, 2023; Pan et al, 2022). Tables 8.9 to 8.13 and Figure 8.10 outline the important practice points for skin care in relation to assessment, risk and prevention/management of pressure sores and wounds. Even the sickest infant requires their basic hygiene needs to be attended to, which is an ideal time to assess skin integrity and to encourage participation in care.

Table 8.9 Neonatal skin assessment

- Check for skin integrity at birth and regularly thereafter in line with timing of care. Observe colour, appearance, level of moisture/dryness and if skin is intact.

- Observe for specific risks: skin oedema, poor skin perfusion, muscle relaxants and gestational age – the premature infant has immature and more fragile skin.

→

Table 8.9 (cont.)

- Pay attention to vulnerable sites – eg nappy and umbilical area, lines, tubes and/or adhesives (nasal CPAP, endotracheal tube (lips), gastric tubes), probe sites (eg saturation, transcutaneous), IV and arterial line sites. Observe for areas of trauma and increased skin vulnerability: epidermal stripping, tearing from adhesive and friction, contact injury (chemicals, moisture, irritants), nappy dermatitis and ischaemic injury.

- Assess and follow specific instructions according to risk and/or from specialist/ tissue viability nurse in the presence of surgical wounds.

- A skin viability assessment tool can be used – for example, the Neonatal Tissue Viability Assessment Tool based on the adapted Braden Q scale (Ashworth and Briggs, 2011) or the Adapted Glamorgan Pressure Ulcer Risk Assessment Scale (HealthCare Improvement Scotland (HIS), 2020).

- Importantly, pay particular attention to neonates with black and brown skin tones when assessing skin colour as it may be more challenging to identify compromise (Carter et al, 2023; Pan et al, 2022).

- Assessment: No/Low risk/At risk/High risk/Very high risk. (Based on various criteria such as intensity/duration of pressure, skin structure and presence of risk factors – activity, sensory perception, moisture, friction, nutrition, tissue perfusion and oxygenation.)

 For skin assessment tools in full and further details, including assessment of ethnically diverse neonates, see the web companion.

 Stop and think

Regular skin assessment including any areas of concern, risk or actual skin damage must be incorporated into an infant's care plan. Remember to consider skin tone – refer to the guidance by Mukwende et al (2020), *Mind the Gap*, on assessing different skin colours/tones.

⊞ Table 8.10 Nursing actions according to skin viability risk

Category	Suggested action
Not at risk/low risk	Continue to reassess daily and every time condition changes.
At risk	Inspect skin with all care procedures. Relieve pressure by regular position changes. Resite monitoring probes frequently, use protective dressings under cannulas and endotracheal tubes or nasal CPAP fixation tapes, ensuring these are not too tight and make frequent checks on at-risk areas.

Category	Suggested action
High risk	Inspect skin with each repositioning/care as above. Use adjuncts to relieve pressure – eg gel mattress. Seek advice from tissue viability nurse.
Very high risk	Inspect skin at least hourly if condition allows. Conduct more regular probe changes. Avoid adhesive tapes. Refer to tissue viability nurse.

 Check local guidance

Check local guidance on skin viability risk and necessary actions.

ASSESSMENT OF SKIN AND RISK OF PRESSURE ULCERS

- Perform skin assessment (see Table 8.9).

PREVENTION

- Take note of skin changes in the occipital area, ears and heels.
- Note blanching erythema or skin discolouration.
- Reposition infant if required or risks are identified.
- Relieve pressure on the scalp/head, heels, ears and knees if prone.
- Consider pressure redistributing device pillows for infants at risk.

MANAGEMENT

- Document the surface area and depth of any pressure area.
- Categorise any pressure area using the European Pressure Ulcer Advisory Panel (EPUAP, 2024) classification system (grades 1 to 4).
- Assess fluid balance and ensure hydration is optimised.
- Refer to Table 8.11 and seek advice from the tissue viability nurse.

 Figure 8.10 Prevention and management of pressure ulcers in the infant (Adapted from National Institute for Health and Care Excellence (NICE), 2014)

Stop and think

Infants considered to be 'at risk' of pressure ulcers are identified after assessment using clinical judgement and/or an agreed risk assessment tool (NICE, 2014), taking into account all skin tones for all neonates for inclusive practice.

⊞ Table 8.11 Neonatal wound assessment

Classification of wound can be undertaken by observing the colour, which indicates the stage of wound healing and/or any presence of infection.

Wound colour

Pink: epithelialising – new growth of skin

Red: granulating – new vascular connective tissue

Yellow: slough (dead cells)

Green/yellow: infected

Black: necrotic tissue

Wound site	Document site(s) and indicate on care plan where the wound is.
Wound size	Width, breadth and depth – record all.
	Possible drawing in care plan of shape and size.
Thickness/depth	Partial thickness – damage to epidermis and dermis.
	Full thickness – also involves subcutaneous tissue and below.
Exudate	Serous fluid, blood or pus.
Odour	None to mild to obvious.
Skin integrity	Surrounding skin – assess colour, moisture, breakdown, oedema, pain, rash, skin changes and infection.
Skin maturity	Gestation – observe presence of translucency, friability and integrity.
Pain	Present all the time or at dressing change only.

(Steen et al, 2020; August et al, 2022)

Check local guidance

Check local guidance on wound assessment.

 Table 8.12 Neonatal wound care

- Causes of wounds in the infant: trauma (epidermal stripping, tearing), surgical incisions, contact excoriation (chemicals, moisture, urine/stool), extravasation, thermal injury, pressure ulcers, CPAP prongs/mask, ischemia and congenital (epidermolysis bullosa, gastroschisis, myelomeningocele).

- Is it clean and dry? **No action required**. Superficial wounds can be exposed to air.

- Or is the wound breaking down/discharge present? **Refer and seek advice from wound care specialist/tissue viability nurse (TVN)**

- Devise plan of care and frequency of dressing change with TVN and document. Review wound appearance and care with each dressing change until healing has been achieved.

- Protect any wound from trauma with non-adherent dressing/covering, one that maintains an ideal environment for wound healing (low adherent, vapour permeable).

- Deeper, more significant wounds that are granulating heal better with moist wound healing/dressing to promote the optimum environment for epithelialisation and growth of new skin tissue and the prevention of trauma from the wound drying out.

- Dressing choice will depend on type and depth of wound and level of exudate. Hydrocolloid sheets are self-adhesive, absorb fluid and are impermeable to bacteria. They may include a soft, non-adherent silicone layer (pink). Other options are an amorphous hydrogel with semi-permeable non-occlusive dressing (red) or a hydrocolloid fibrous dressing with foam (for infected wounds).

- Wound cleansing may be necessary in the presence of debris, bacteria or necrosis. Routine cleansing of all wounds however is not necessary.

(Steen et al, 2020)

 Stop and think

Whatever the cause, the aims of wound care are the same: to protect the wound area, to promote optimum healing and resumed skin integrity, to prevent breakdown and, if necessary, to provide gentle cleansing and treatment in the presence of infection.

Table 8.13 Hygiene care in the neonatal unit

- Gather all items required including gloves and a disposal bag.

- **Nappy care:** Change nappy at intervals according to the infant's condition and tolerance. Use water only. Observe nappy area closely; if rash is present, expose if possible.

- **Bathing:** In special care. Time according to gestation, weight and temperature.

- **Top and tail:** Face and nappy area only – most common in intensive care.

- **Eye care:** Not routine. Use sterile gauze, one piece for each eye, and using sterile water sweep inwards to outwards, discarding each gauze piece with each sweep.

- **Mouth care:** Use cotton buds to clean mouth with water and keep lips/tongue moist.

- **Umbilical cord care:** In the healthy, term, near term or healthy preterm infants at birth, evidence supports leaving the cord for at least one minute prior to clamping and cutting. Once clamped and cut, the cord is kept clean and observed until the stump separates. In the sick or high-risk infant who requires admission to neonatal care, the cord is clamped and cut immediately, leaving a long stump which may be catheterised. Only use water to clean the area around the stump. Ensure the stump dries up and separates by 5–15 days. If there is any redness or discharge, send swab and refer for possible antibiotics. See also Chapter 2.

(NICE, 2021a; Johnson, 2016)

 Standard precautions alert

Effective hygiene care in the neonatal unit is essential to limit the risk of infection in vulnerable, small and/or sick infants, timed according to their needs and stress tolerance levels. Importantly, involve parents in this aspect of care as much as possible or as much as they prefer.

INFECTION IN THE NEONATAL UNIT

Immaturity and illness make infants vulnerable to infection, which is associated with increased mortality, increased length of stay and healthcare costs, and risk of neurodevelopmental disability among survivors (Johnson et al, 2021). It is therefore imperative that measures are taken to prevent it. Standard precautions must be always adhered to, including hand hygiene, protective clothing, sharps and waste disposal, management of care equipment and environment, and the safe care of linen including uniforms. It is worth reiterating that thorough handwashing is vital. The World Health Organization's 'Five moments for hand hygiene' should be followed (before touching a patient, before procedures, after contact with body fluids, after touching a patient or their surroundings). Table 8.14 outlines neonatal infection, assessment and the septic screen.

 Table 8.14 Understanding neonatal infection and the septic screen

Risk factors and clinical signs

- Kaiser Permanente Risk Calculator may be utilised and is endorsed by NICE (2021b).

Early onset infection (within 72 hours)

- Identify maternal signs: fever, high C-reactive protein (CRP), offensive amniotic fluid, previous infections and need for antibiotics.

- Clinical signs range from non-specific or vague symptoms to a hemodynamic collapse. Early symptoms may include irritability, lethargy or poor feeding.

- Neonatal 'red flags' – risk of group B Streptococcus (GBS), prolonged rupture of membranes, preterm birth, fever (38 degrees Celsius), respiratory distress, need for ventilation, poor perfusion/shock.

Late onset infection (after 72 hours)

- Central lines, invasive procedures, ventilation, steroid therapy, poor nutrition, poor skin integrity, poor hygiene and handwashing practices, cross-infection.

Septic screen

- Clinical assessment – see above.

- Haematological markers – culture, full blood count/white cell count, platelets, clotting, lactate, CRP.

- Swabs.

- Urine.

- If strong suspicion of neurological involvement – lumbar puncture.

Antibiotics

Empiric treatment with IV antibiotics should be started as soon as sepsis is clinically suspected and always within 60 minutes of the decision to treat (NICE, 2021b). The length of course will depend on clinical and laboratory findings. For infants who require an antibiotic course longer than 36–48 hours, the gentamicin level will be checked prior to the second or third dose (refer to local guidance) (NICE, 2021b). In infants with RDS, antibiotics should be used judiciously and stopped early when sepsis is ruled out (Sweet et al, 2023).

Stop and think

In any infant that deteriorates, infection should always be considered as a potential diagnosis and a septic screen commenced as soon as possible.

CARE OF THE HOSPITALISED JAUNDICED INFANT

Physiological jaundice is usually a mild, transient and self-limiting condition and resolves without treatment (see Chapter 2). However, it is imperative to distinguish this from 'pathological jaundice' as severe hyperbilirubinemia can cause bilirubin-induced neurological dysfunction (BIND) and, if not treated adequately, may lead to encephalopathy (Ullah et al, 2016). Unconjugated hyperbilirubinemia is the most common type of jaundice; however, a conjugated form can present, which is pathological and signifies an underlying medical or surgical cause. The main treatment is phototherapy, which converts unconjugated bilirubin to a conjugated, safe form that can be excreted, and is started when the bilirubin values exceed the 'threshold'. Chapter 2 introduces neonatal jaundice; the current chapter covers jaundice types, measuring bilirubin, methods of phototherapy, related care and a brief introduction to exchange blood transfusions, which are required when phototherapy is no longer effective as a treatment option (Tables 8.15 to 8.18 and Figures 8.11 to 8.12).

 Stop and think

Refer to the NICE guidance on neonatal jaundice for treatment threshold graphs for different gestational ages. Premature infants have a lowered threshold for starting treatment (NICE, 2010).

⊞ Table 8.15 Types of neonatal jaundice

Jaundice type	Onset/timing	Type of bilirubin
Physiological	After day 3 to day 7 approximately	Unconjugated
Pathological	Within the first 24 hours	Unconjugated
Prolonged	Persists past the usual 7–10 days period	Conjugated or unconjugated

⊞ Table 8.16 Assessing for the presence of jaundice

Clinical observation	Transcutaneous (TcB) (skin)	Serum bilirubin (SBR)
View the infant naked in good, natural light. Observe the eye sclera, oral mucosa (eg lips, tongue, gums) and blanched skin (eg of nail beds when gently pressed) for the presence of yellow discolouration. Do not solely rely on skin assessment as this does not identify visible jaundice in neonates with black or brown skin tones (NHS Race and Health Observatory, 2023). This method however should not be relied on solely.	Sternum (and sometimes the forehead) site for application of non-invasive transcutaneous probe for near term infants *after* the first 24 hours and for infants born >35 weeks' gestation. Readings above 250 micromols/L are unreliable and so SBR should be used in this situation (NICE, 2010).	Use when TcB method is not available OR for infants less than 24 hours old, where visible jaundice is present and for any infant born at less than 35 weeks' gestation. For jaundice in the first 24 hours, SBR should be done within two hours. Use SBR for any infant where bilirubin is above treatment threshold.

 Table 8.17 Prolonged jaundice screen

Blood tests

- Total and conjugated serum bilirubin – a 'split bili' blood test differentiates between the two types of bilirubin.
- Full blood count, blood group, direct antibody test and urine culture.
- Liver function tests.
- Thyroxine and thyroid-stimulating hormone.
- Galactosaemia screen.

Urine

- Microscopy, culture and sensitivity.
- Reducing sugars (eg loss of galactose).
- Look for dark urine that stains the nappy.

Stool

- Stool specimen in an opaque pot – look for pale chalky stools.

Other

- Ensure that routine metabolic screening has been performed.
- Infection screen including congenital infection and hepatitis.
- Follow expert advice about care for infants with a conjugated bilirubin level greater than 25 micromols/litre.

(NICE, 2010)

Stop and think

Prolonged jaundice may be indicative of a serious disease that requires treatment. Therefore, assessment and monitoring are vital.

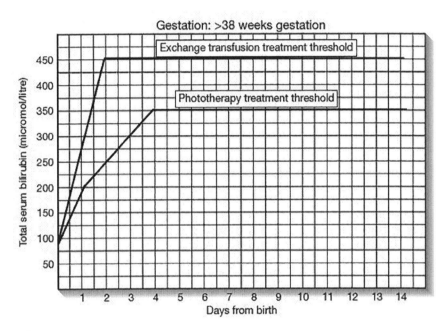

Figure 8.11 Treatment threshold graph for phototherapy and exchange transfusion

Table 8.18 Phototherapy devices

Conventional	Fibreoptic
Light source delivered via halogen bulb, fluorescent lamps or light-emitting diodes. Distance of light varies depending on model: range 25–50 cm from infant.	Light is passed through a fibreoptic bundle and is placed next to the skin – eg biliblanket or bed/mattress.

Combination

- Use both conventional and fibreoptic together to increase irradiance of light.
- Double or triple phototherapy can be used to increase effectiveness.

Requirements of effective phototherapy

- An effective spectrum of light – in white or blue range (intensity 400–520 nm).
- Sufficient irradiance of light – a measure of the amount of light reaching the skin.
- Maximum expose of skin surface area to the phototherapy light.
- Metalloporphyrins may be used as a preventative measure.

 Stop and think

Double or triple phototherapy should be attempted where high levels of SBR (above the treatment threshold) are present to avoid an exchange transfusion being administered.

Neonatal exchange transfusions

Neonatal exchange blood transfusion is a specialist procedure with associated risks and is now infrequently performed in most neonatal units, mainly because of the reduction in haemolytic disease of the newborn (HDN) following routine antenatal anti-D prophylaxis for D-negative women. It must take place in an intensive care setting, with intensive physiological and biochemical monitoring carried out by staff trained in the procedure following written informed parental consent (New et al, 2011). The aim of the dilutional exchange is to reduce the packed cell volume (PCV) to 50–55% in the case of symptomatic polycythaemia. The infant should be admitted to high dependency or intensive care and cardiopulmonary monitoring commenced.

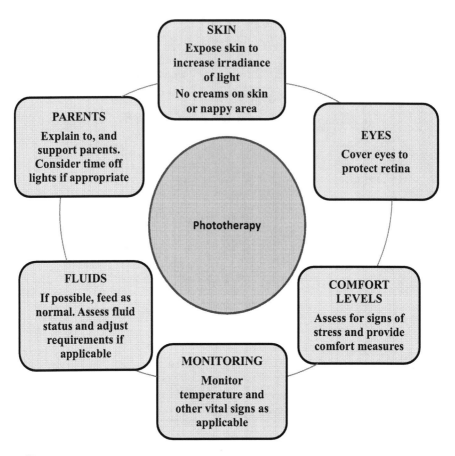

 Figure 8.12 Care of the infant receiving phototherapy. The aim is to provide a balance between normalising care and reducing bilirubin levels as soon as possible

The introduction of neonatal community outreach services allows some areas to offer home phototherapy for infants meeting a set criterion.

See the web companion for a glossary specific to this chapter.

📍 *Check local variations and guidance alert*

The space below can be used to record any notes, local variations and practice points specific to your own unit.

REFERENCES

Alsweiler, J M, Kuschel, C A and Bloomfield, F H (2007) Survey of the Management of Neonatal Hyperglycaemia in Australasia. *Journal of Paediatrics and Child Health*, 43(9): 632–5.

Ashworth, C and Briggs, L (2011) Design and Implementation of a Neonatal Tissue Viability Assessment Tool on the Newborn Intensive Care Unit. *Infant*, 7(6): 191–4.

August, D, Kandasamy, Y, Ray, R, New, K and Lindsay, D (2022) Evaluation of the Consistency of Neonatal Skin Injury Assessment Using Clinical Images and the Metric and Graduated Colour Tool. *Journal of Tissue Viability*, 31(3): 395–403.

Beardsall, K (2021) Hyperglycaemia in the Newborn Infant: Physiology Verses Pathology. *Frontiers in Pediatrics*, 9: 641306.

British Association of Perinatal Medicine (BAPM) (2019) Improving Normothermia in Very Preterm Infants: A Quality Improvement Toolkit. [online] Available at: www.bapm.org/pages/105-normothermia-toolkit (accessed 31 October 2023).

British Association of Perinatal Medicine (BAPM) (2024) *Identification and Management of Neonatal Hypoglycaemia in the Full-Term Infant: A BAPM Framework for Practice*. [online] Available at: www.bapm.org/resources/identification-and-management-of-neonatal-hypoglycaemia-in-the-full-term-infant-birth-72-hours (accessed 28 January 2024).

Carter, B M, Newberry, D and Leonard, C (2023) Color Does Matter: Nursing Assessment of Varying Skin Tones/Pigmentation. *Advances in Neonatal Care*, 23(6): 525–31.

Cherian, S, Morris, I, Evans, J and Kotecha, S (2014) Oxygen Therapy in Preterm Infants. *Paediatric Respiratory Reviews*, 15(2): 135–41.

Cranmer, H (2022) Neonatal Hypoglycaemia. [online] Available at: https://emedicine.medscape.com/article/802334-overview?form=fpf (accessed 24 January 2024).

Embleton, N D, Moltu, S J, Lapillonne, A et al (2023) Enteral Nutrition in Preterm Infants (2022): A Position Paper from the ESPGHAN Committee on Nutrition and Invited Experts. *Journal of Pediatric Gastroenterology and Nutrition*, 76(2): 248–68.

European Pressure Ulcer Advisory Panel (EPUAP) and National Pressure Ulcer Advisory Panel (NPUAP) (2024) *Pressure Ulcer Prevention: Quick Reference Guide*. [online] Available at: www.epuap.org/wp-content/uploads/2016/10/quick-reference-guide-digital-npuap-epuap-pppia-jan2016.pdf (accessed 28 January 2024).

Gardner, S L, Carter, B S, Enzman-Hines, M and Niermeyer, S (2020) *Merenstein & Gardner's Handbook of Neonatal Intensive Care: An Interprofessional Approach.* 9th ed. St. Louis, MO: Elsevier.

Glass, L and Valdez, A (2021) Preterm Infant Incubator Humidity Levels: A Systematic Review. *Advances in Neonatal Care,* 21(4): 297–307.

HealthCare Improvement Scotland (HIS) (2020) Paediatric Risk Assessment Tool. [online] Available at: www.healthcareimprovementscotland.org/our_work/patient_safety/tissue_viability_resources/paediatric_glamorgan_tool.aspx (accessed 31 October 2023).

Jochum, F, Moltu, S J, Senterre, T, Nomayo, A, Goulet, O and Iacobelli, S (2018) ESPGHAN/ESPEN/ESPR/CSPEN Guidelines on Pediatric Parenteral Nutrition: Fluid and Electrolytes. *Clinical Nutrition,* 37(6): 2344–53.

Johnson, D E (2016) Extremely Preterm Infant Skin Care. *Advances in Neonatal Care,* 16(5): 26–32.

Johnson, J, Akinboyo, I C and Schaffzin, J K (2021) Infection Prevention in the Neonatal Intensive Care Unit. *Clinics in Perinatology,* 48(2): 413–29.

Lyu, Y, Shah, P S, Ye X Y and Canadian Neonatal Network (2015) Association between Admission Temperature and Mortality and Major Morbidity in Preterm Infants Born at Fewer Than 33 Weeks' Gestation. *JAMA Pediatrics,* 169(4).

McCall, E M, Alderdice, F, Vohara, S et al (2018) Interventions to Prevent Hypothermia at Birth in Preterm and/or Low Birthweight Infants. *Cochrane Database of Systematic Reviews,* 2.

Moss, C R (2022) Fluid and Electrolyte Management in the Neonate: Sodium and Chloride. *Neonatal Network,* 41(3): 137–44.

Mukwende, M, Tamony, P and Turner, M (2020) *Mind the Gap: A Handbook of Clinical Signs in Black and Brown Skin.* London: St George's University of London.

National Health Service (NHS) Race and Health Observatory (2023) Review of Neonatal Assessment and Practice in Black, Asian and Minority Ethnic Newborns: Exploring the Apgar Score, the Detection of Cyanosis and Jaundice. [online] Available at: www.nhsrho.org/research/review-of-neonatal-assessment-and-practice-in-black-asian-and-minority-ethnic-newborns-exploring-the-apgar-score-the-detection-of-cyanosis-and-jaundice (accessed 28 January 2024).

National Institute for Health and Care Excellence (NICE) (2010) Jaundice in Newborn Babies Under 28 Days. Clinical Guideline [CG98]. [online] Available at: www.nice.org.uk/guidance/CG98 (accessed 31 October 2023).

National Institute for Health and Care Excellence (NICE) (2014) Pressure Ulcers: Prevention and Management. Clinical Guideline [CG179]. [online] Available at: www.nice.org.uk/guidance/cg179 (accessed 31 October 2023).

National Institute for Health and Care Excellence (NICE) (2021a) Postnatal Care. NICE Guideline [NG194]. [online] Available at: www.nice.org.uk/guidance/ng194 (accessed 31 October 2023).

National Institute for Health and Care Excellence (NICE) (2021b) Neonatal Infection: Antibiotics for Prevention and Treatment. NICE Guideline [NG195]. [online] Available at: www.nice.org.uk/guidance/ng195 (accessed 31 October 2023).

New, K, Flenady, V and Davies, M W (2011) Transfer of Preterm Infants from Incubator to Open Cot at Lower Versus Higher Body Weight. *Cochrane Database of Systematic Reviews*, 9: CD004214.

Oranges, T, Dini, V and Romanelli, M (2015) Skin Physiology of the Neonate and Infant: Clinical Implications. *Advances in Wound Care*, 4(10): 587–95.

Pan, C X, Yang, K and Nambudiri, V E (2022) Assessment of the Representation of Black, Indigenous and People of Colour in Dermatology Clinical Practice Guidelines. *British Journal of Dermatology*, 187(3): 443–5.

Steen, E H, Wang, X, Boochoon, K S et al (2020) Wound Healing and Wound Care in Neonates: Current Therapies and Novel Options. *Advances in Skin & Wound Care*, 33(6): 294–300.

Sweet, D G, Carnielli, V P, Greisen, G et al (2023) European Consensus Guidelines on the Management of Respiratory Distress Syndrome: 2022 Update. *Neonatology*, 120(1): 3–23.

Tume, L N, Valla, F V, Joosten, K, Jotterand Chaparro, C, Latten, L, Marino, L V, Macleod, I, Moullet, C, Pathan, N, Rooze, S, van Rosmalen, J and Verbruggen, S C A T (2020) Nutritional Support for Children During Critical Illness: European Society of Pediatric and Neonatal Intensive Care (ESPNIC) Metabolism, Endocrine and Nutrition Section Position Statement and Clinical Recommendations. *Intensive Care Medicine*, 46(3): 411–25.

Turnbull, V and Petty, J (2013) Evidence-based Thermal Care of Low Birthweight Neonates: Part One. *Nursing Children and Young People*, 25(2): 18–22.

UK Resuscitation Council (2021) Newborn Resuscitation and Support of Transition of Infants at Birth Guidelines. [online] Available at: www.resus.org.uk/library/2021-resuscitation-guidelines/newborn-resuscitation-and-support-transition-infants-birth (accessed 28 January 2024).

Ullah, S, Rahman, K and Hedayati, M (2016) Hyperbilirubinemia in Neonates: Types, Causes, Clinical Examinations, Preventive Measures and Treatments: A Narrative Review Article. *Iranian Journal of Public Health*, 45(5): 558–68.

UNICEF (2016) Baby Friendly Guidelines. [online] Available at: www.unicef.org.uk/babyfriendly (accessed 5 December 2023).

Wood, T, Johnson, M, Temples, T and Bordelon, C (2022) Thermoneutral Environment for Neonates: Back to the Basics. *Neonatal Network*, 41(5): 289–96.

9 Developmentally supportive care to promote well-being in the neonatal setting

Katy Moss, Julia Petty, Michelle Scott and Melanie Carpenter

INTRODUCTION

Developmental care in the neonatal unit is an area concerned with promoting the well-being of the neonate by implementing developmentally supportive measures and promoting an environment that minimises stress (Williams et al, 2018). Developmental care promotes positive neonatal neurodevelopment and behavioural outcomes involving many important components (Altimier and Phillips, 2013). This includes positive touch, providing appropriate sound levels and lighting, careful positioning and handling, promotion of sleep, minimising stress and pain, optimising nutrition and managing skin integrity, all emphasising the need to treat the neonate according to their behavioural and physiological cues. Parents should be involved with all aspects of the neonate's care; we must look at the neonate and family as a whole and promote individualised, inclusive and culturally appropriate family integrated care. Preterm neonates who receive consistent individualised developmentally supportive care from birth demonstrate fewer behavioural stress cues and improved neurodevelopmental outcomes (O'Brien et al, 2018; Séassau et al, 2023). This chapter addresses the important elements of developmental care; namely, an overview of the concept (Figure 9.1), seven key components (Table 9.1), principles of good positioning (Table 9.2), recognising and minimising stress (Table 9.3), environmental care (Figures 9.2 and 9.3), pain management (Figures 9.4 and 9.5) and skin-to-skin care (Figures 9.6 to 9.8).

Chapter learning objectives

By the end of this chapter you will:

✓ be able to understand the importance of developmental care and how it can improve neonatal outcomes;

✓ be able to recognise good positioning and handling to optimise comfort and well-being and minimise stress in the neonate.

Critical thinking points

- How can different stresses affect neonatal development and outcomes and why?

- What is the importance of involving parents/caregivers early in the neonate's care journey?

 The areas covered in this chapter closely interrelate to optimising the comfort, well-being and outcomes of neonates within a family perspective; refer also to Chapter 12.

 See the web companion for supplementary information relating to the topics throughout this chapter.

Stop and think

Developmental care is part of the holistic management of any neonate, however sick or preterm, with individualised and inclusive care tailored to their needs.

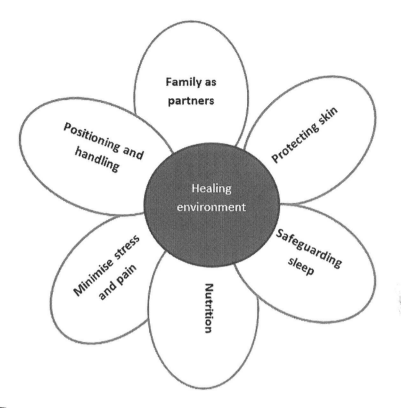

↗ Figure 9.1 Neonatal integrative developmental care model
(Altimier and Philips, 2013)

⊞ Table 9.1 Seven principles of neonatal developmental care

Healing environment	• Create an environment that reduces stress and extra stimuli.
	• Noise reduction – excessive noise can affect the neurodevelopment of the neonate, especially preterm.
	• Excessive light or dark – promote quiet times and day and night cycles.
	• There is a relationship between the environment and brain development. As a result of excessive stimuli, neurons may form alternative pathways between the cerebral cortex and the brainstem (Aita et al, 2021).
Minimising stress and pain	• Premature and sick term infants regularly experience painful and stressful procedures.
	• Use appropriate pain relief, pharmacological or non-pharmacological.
	• Stress and pain have similar physiological and behavioural responses in preterm infants due to their immaturity; it is important to observe babies' cues.

→

Table 9.1 (cont.)

Partnering with families	• Bonding starts early in a pregnancy and in the event of a preterm birth, this process may be disrupted. Separation can affect the normal physical contact and emotional closeness. It is important to support parents/caregivers to maintain this bond using skin to skin. • Support parents/caregivers to be involved in cares.
Protecting skin	• Term or preterm babies are at risk of skin integrity deterioration during their stay in the neonatal unit due to the intense light, frequent touch and diagnostic and therapeutic applications that occur within the unit. • Use appropriate wipes, tape etc. • Reposition in a timely manner – look for pressure marks (redness) on knees, elbows, back, ears, nose and face, being mindful of skin tone according to ethnicity.
Positioning and handling	• Poor positioning can result in causing discomfort, skin breakdown and poor muscle development. Increased handling can enhance stress factors which can affect heart rate, O_2 levels and breathing. • Use good positioning aids to promote sleep and appropriate positions.
Optimising nutrition	• Nutrition is a very important part of a neonate's development. It provides the building blocks for growth and brain development. • Nutrition also promotes immunity, neurodevelopment and decreases hospital stay.
Safeguarding sleep	• Sleep promotes maturation of the central nervous system, memory and learning; it helps maintain energy and promotes growth. • Minimise cares, handling, noise and overstimulation to protect sleeping, which then protects the brain (Aita et al, 2021).

(Altimier and Philips, 2013)

 Stop and think

Developmental care involves a range of areas that combine to create an individualised plan to optimise all aspects of neonatal care. By involving parents and the whole family we can support the neurodevelopment of our patients by improving and supporting bonding and growth (Petty and van den Hoogen, 2022).

POSITIONING THE INFANT

Another aim is to position the neonate appropriately and comfortably while supporting their limbs and head to avoid any short- or long-term effects to the skin or muscular system (Pineda et al, 2014). Appropriate positioning of the neonate serves as a specific example of how care can be developmentally supportive.

 Table 9.2 Positioning sick and preterm neonates

Neonates should be positioned with:

- ✓ symmetrical postures;
- ✓ flexion of limbs;
- ✓ shoulder and hip flexion and adduction;
- ✓ hands near face;
- ✓ neutral alignment of ankles and hips;
- ✓ neutral alignment of head and neck whenever possible;
- ✓ the use of swaddling or nesting to provide boundaries.

(European Foundation for the Care of the Newborn Infant (EFCNI), 2021a)

The supine position

The supine position (ie lying on the back) is often used if neonates are unstable and need to be observed regularly. It facilitates access to the neonate to initiate procedures if necessary. In the neonatal unit, placing them in a more upright position can help facilitate chest expansion. The supine position is also recommended for use at home to ensure safe sleep.

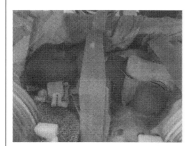 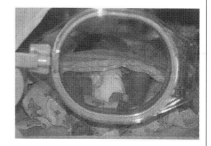

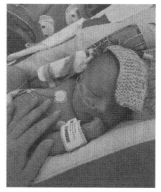

→

Table 9.2 (cont.)

The prone position

The prone position (lying on the tummy/breast) may improve oxygen saturation, respiratory function (Ballout et al, 2017), digestion and sleep. Neonates may lose less heat and energy. However, this position should only be used when the neonate is monitored continuously and should not be used at home due to the risk of sudden infant death syndrome (SIDS).

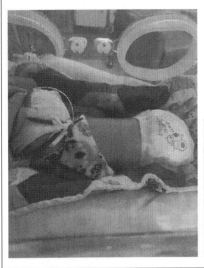
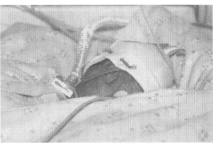

The lateral position

The lateral position (lying on one side) supports a flexed position with bended arms and legs and allows the neonate to adjust their own position. Usually, shoulders are rounded and relaxed, legs are bent with boundaries and hands can reach the mouth and face more easily. This position is often used to reduce stress during cares (eg mouth care, nappy change or tube feeding).

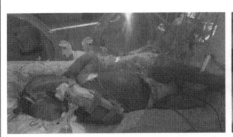
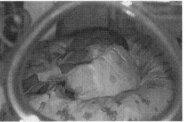

Stop and think

Recognition of behavioural cues during periods of handling informs carers when neonates become stressed. Even the most basic of care procedures can cause physiological stress and therefore a 'time-out' period should be initiated.

 ## Standard precautions

Remember infection control when positioning.

 ## Stop and think

Once a neonate's condition has improved prior to discharge, remember to always place the neonate supine, as per the guidelines for the prevention of SIDS.

Table 9.3 Neonatal stress cues and interventions

Relaxed	Stress cues	Interventions
• Normal and regular heart rate	• Changes in skin colour	• Practising skin-to-skin care
• Gentle, regular breathing	• Low or high heart rate	• Breastfeeding or providing mother's milk
• Normal oxygen saturation	• Rapid breathing; irregular breathing with pauses	• Placing the hands on the baby's head and lower back or feet: containment holding
• Digesting food without discomfort	• Lower oxygen saturation	
	• Vomiting (throwing up) or gagging	• Placing the baby in a nest (rolled-up sheets to form boundaries around the baby)
• Gentle movements	• Hiccups	
	• Sounds of regurgitation	• Comfortable positioning

→

Table 9.3 (cont.)

Relaxed	Stress cues	Interventions
• Firm muscle tone (but not too tight)	• Choking, burping	• Avoiding direct light exposure
• Arms and legs folded towards body	• Frantic movements, tremors	• Maintaining low levels of ambient light
• Hands resting on face or head	• Low muscle tone; loss of energy	• Adapting the medical and care procedures to the sleep–wake-cycles of the baby slow the pace of what you are doing or give the neonate a break if stress signs are noted
• Hands and feet brought together	• Fingers or toes stretched wide; tight fists	
• Relaxed face	• Arching and stiffness	
• Sucking	• Straining	
• Shiny alert eyes or eyes closed	• Grimacing	• Optimising pain management
	• Yawning	
	• Looking away, staring, panicked look, gazing	• Encourage self-regulatory behaviours: hand to mouth, grasping, sucking and hand clasping
	• Crying	

(Adapted from EFCNI, 2021b)

 Also refer to the section on pain management in this chapter.

 Check local guidance

Ensure individual unit policies are checked and advice sought from developmental and environmental care experts within the multi-disciplinary team in relation to best practices.

ENVIRONMENTAL CARE

Developmental care includes management of the *surroundings* within the neonatal unit, incorporating the acoustic, light and thermal environment. The potentially harmful effects of the environment on the preterm neonate are well documented (Orsi et al, 2017). Figure 9.2 illustrates a covered incubator to minimise light and disturbances, while Figure 9.3 provides an overview of how to optimise the neonatal environment.

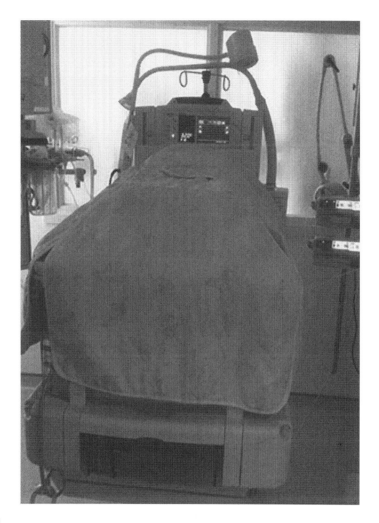

 Figure 9.2 Incubator with cover

> ### 🖐 *Stop and think*
>
> Exposure to inappropriate noise levels may cause physiological insta-
> bility, agitation and disrupted sleep patterns. The aim of environmen-
> tal care is to mimic the uterine environment, promote physical stability,
> avoid hypoxia and support organised sleep patterns and circadian
> rhythms (EFCNI, 2021a).

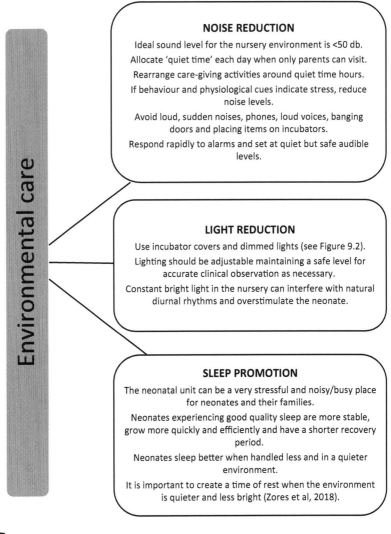

NOISE REDUCTION

Ideal sound level for the nursery environment is <50 db.

Allocate 'quiet time' each day when only parents can visit.

Rearrange care-giving activities around quiet time hours.

If behaviour and physiological cues indicate stress, reduce noise levels.

Avoid loud, sudden noises, phones, loud voices, banging doors and placing items on incubators.

Respond rapidly to alarms and set at quiet but safe audible levels.

LIGHT REDUCTION

Use incubator covers and dimmed lights (see Figure 9.2).

Lighting should be adjustable maintaining a safe level for accurate clinical observation as necessary.

Constant bright light in the nursery can interfere with natural diurnal rhythms and overstimulate the neonate.

SLEEP PROMOTION

The neonatal unit can be a very stressful and noisy/busy place for neonates and their families.

Neonates experiencing good quality sleep are more stable, grow more quickly and efficiently and have a shorter recovery period.

Neonates sleep better when handled less and in a quieter environment.

It is important to create a time of rest when the environment is quieter and less bright (Zores et al, 2018).

Environmental care

Figure 9.3 Optimising the neonatal environment

PAIN MANAGEMENT AND ASSESSMENT

Neonates in hospital may experience pain from a variety of sources, including diagnostic/therapeutic interventions or because of illness, and exhibit a range of pain cues (Figure 9.4). Assessing neonates for pain is paramount so that adequate treatment can be provided. The prevention of pain is important not only because it is an ethical expectation of care but also because repeated painful exposures can have deleterious consequences. A variety of neonatal pain assessment tools exist that aim to assess physiological and behavioural responses to being exposed to noxious stimuli (Perry et al, 2018). Tools can serve to aid the clinical assessment of pain to ensure consistency between staff and carers. There are common elements between different tools – see the web companion for examples. Selection of a pain assessment tool is dependent on individual neonatal unit choice and local guidance/preference.

Pain management is an essential component of neonatal care to promote optimum well-being and relieve stress in both the neonate and family, both physiological and psychological. An individual approach should be used for each neonate using a standardised approach and a combination of non-pharmacological and pharmacological pain-relieving interventions (Figure 9.5), along with a greater active engagement of parents in the pain care for their preterm infant (Campbell-Yeo et al, 2022).

 See Chapter 5 and refer to the web companion site for further detail on, and examples of, pain assessment tools.

Physiological cues
Respiration – apnoea
Heart rate – fluctuating or tachycardic
Saturations – desaturating
Blood pressure – hypotensive or hypertensive or normal
Colour – pale, dusky

Behavioural cues
Posture and tone – tense, fists clenched, trunk guarded, limbs adducted, head and shoulders resist positioning and/or extended, trunk rigid, limbs abducted
Sleep pattern – is the neonate very agitated or withdrawn, easily woken, restless, squirming, no clear sleep/wake cycles, eye aversion 'shut out'?
Expression – is there a grimace, deep brow furrows, eyes tightly closed, pupils dilated or frown present, shallow brow furrows, eyes lightly closed?
Cry – when disturbed, does not settle after handling, loud, whimper, whining

Biochemical cues
Blood glucose
Blood gases – drops in PaO$_2$

Sources of pain
Surgery
Heel lance
Venepuncture
Tape removal
Moving and handling
Nasogastric tube insertion
Eye (ROP) examinations
Chest drain insertion and removal
Intubation
Extravasation injury and other skin trauma

Special considerations
Preterm infants may have an exaggerated response to painful stimuli
A neonate with neurological impairment may not exhibit the usual tachycardic response and facial expression.
Neonates who are receiving muscle-relaxants can only be assessed based on their physiological changes

 Figure 9.4 An overview of neonatal pain sources and cues

Stop and think

Assessment of pain and stress should be carried out in all neonates of any level of dependency. Signs are non-specific and not always obvious, especially in very small, preterm neonates – therefore, interpretation may not be straightforward. Pain assessment should be incorporated into a care plan and be part of holistic, regular assessment along with vital signs and other physiological cues.

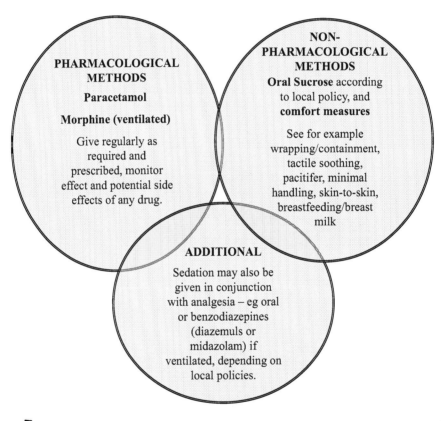

PHARMACOLOGICAL METHODS

Paracetamol

Morphine (ventilated)

Give regularly as required and prescribed, monitor effect and potential side effects of any drug.

NON-PHARMACOLOGICAL METHODS

Oral Sucrose according to local policy, and **comfort measures**

See for example wrapping/containment, tactile soothing, pacitifer, minimal handling, skin-to-skin, breastfeeding/breast milk

ADDITIONAL

Sedation may also be given in conjunction with analgesia – eg oral or benzodiazepines (diazemuls or midazolam) if ventilated, depending on local policies.

 Figure 9.5 Neonatal pain management – overview

◉ Check local guidance

Check local guidance for agreed strategies such as the use of sucrose for procedural pain.

Stop and think

A combination of both approaches, pharmacological and non-pharmacological, is preferable rather than relying on just one. Use of sucrose is dependent on the individual unit and if used there will be a policy on how, when and what to administer.

SKIN-TO-SKIN CARE AND DELIVERY ROOM CUDDLES

A related area to developmental care is that of delivery room cuddles (Figure 9.6) and 'Kangaroo care', otherwise called skin-to-skin contact (SSC) (Figures 9.7 and 9.8), which was introduced in Chapters 5 and 6. Early care of infants in the delivery suite or neonatal unit that includes the encouragement of early breastfeeding and skin-to-skin contact has reported benefits, namely, better neonatal thermal control, reduction of stress, improved cardio-respiratory stability and decreased crying (Lee et al, 2022), reduction of procedural pain (Campbell-Yeo et al, 2022) and facilitation of breastfeeding and parental bonding (Siva et al, 2023). Cuddling their baby after birth is instinctive for parents, irrespective of gestation, and facilitation of a first cuddle between parents and their newborn in the delivery room is the ideal way to form an initial physical and psychological bond and for the baby to feel their first embrace (Clarke et al, 2021). Regular skin-to-skin care practice can be undertaken in any part of the neonatal unit; it should be routine care and strongly promoted.

 Stop and think

Skin-to-skin care can be given to any neonate, even those in intensive care if their condition allows, while ensuring family support is given throughout in an inclusive way for all parents. It is important to consider and offer kangaroo care to *both* parents.

DON'T FORGET DELIVERY ROOM CUDDLES

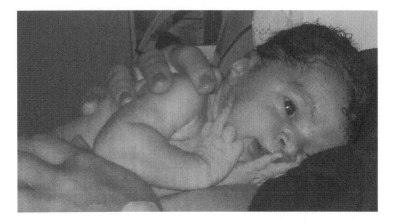

 Figure 9.6 Delivery room cuddle

PREPARATION
Assess readiness of neonate, parents and neonatal staff/unit.
Explain benefits and process to parents. Ensure SSC is part of the developmental care plan.
Secure all tubes and lines. Set up position of chair and any support necessary. Get parent(s) into position. Provide blanket and hat for the infant and check vital signs.

TRANSFER
Remove carefully from incubator with another nurse to hold and lines or tubes if necessary.
Place upright on parent's chest (Figure 9.8), legs and arms flexed, head and neck positioned to ensure open airway. The face may be directed towards parent's face.
Keep neonate against the skin but covered over the back with hat on.

MONITORING
Observe for signs of instability (apnoea, desaturation, drops in central temperature).
Contraindications include any neonate with a chest drain, arterial line, on high frequency ventilation or inhaled nitric oxide or one who has been unstable within the last 24 hours.
Continue with vital sign monitoring including pulse oximetry.
Check temperature regularly according to neonate's gestation and thermal stability.
Assess comfort levels.
Tube feeding can continue.

TRANSFER BACK
Move back to incubator when ready / appropriate as planned.

Figure 9.7 Skin-to-skin care in the neonatal unit

◉ Check local guidance

Check local guidance on any relevant skin-to-skin care policy.

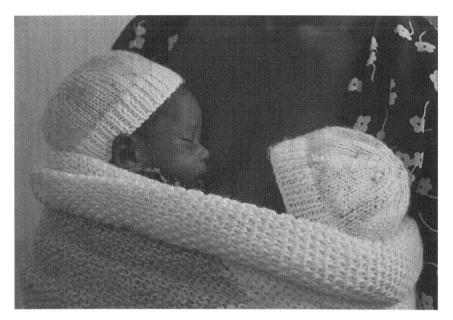

 Figure 9.8 Skin-to-skin care

🖐 Standard precautions alert

Strict infection control measures must be applied to the neonatal environment.

 See Chapter 16 for organisations that support and provide training and resources to promote developmental care.

 See web companion for a glossary specific to this chapter.

Check local variations and guidance alert

The space below can be used to record any notes or local variations and practice points specific to your own unit.

REFERENCES

Aita, M, De Clifford Faugère, G, Lavallée, A, Feeley, N, Stremler, R, Rioux, É and Proulx, M H (2021) Effectiveness of Interventions on Early Neurodevelopment of Preterm Infants: A Systematic Review and Meta-Analysis. *BMC Pediatrics*, 21(1): 1–17.

Altimier, L and Phillips, R M (2013) The Neonatal Integrative Developmental Care Model: Seven Neuroprotective Core Measures for Family-Centered Developmental Care. *Newborn and Infant Nursing Reviews*, 13(1): 9–22.

Ballout, R A, Foster, J P, Kahale, L A and Badr, L (2017) Body Positioning for Spontaneously Breathing Preterm Infants with Apnoea. *Cochrane Database of Syst Rev*, 1: CD004951.

Campbell-Yeo, M, Eriksson, M and Benoit, B (2022) Assessment and Management of Pain in Preterm Infants: A Practice Update. *Children*, 9(2): 244.

Clarke, P, Allen, E, Atuona, S and Cawley, P (2021) Delivery Room Cuddles for Extremely Preterm Babies and Parents: Concept, Practice, Safety, Parental Feedback. *Acta Paediatrica*, 110(5): 1439–49.

European Foundation for the Care of Newborn Infants (EFCNI) (2021a) Positioning. [online] Available at: www.efcni.org/health-topics/in-hospital/developmental-care/positioning (accessed 5 December 2023).

European Foundation for the Care of Newborn Infants (EFCNI) (2021b) Recognising the Baby's Signs. [online] Available at: www.efcni.org/health-topics/in-hospital/recognising-signs (accessed 5 December 2023).

Lee, J, Parikka, V, Lehtonen, L and Soukka, H (2022) Parent-Infant Skin-to-Skin Contact Reduces the Electrical Activity of the Diaphragm and Stabilizes Respiratory Function in Preterm Infants. *Pediatric Research*, 91(5): 1163–7.

O'Brien, K, Robson, K, Bracht, M et al (2018) Effectiveness of Family Integrated Care in Neonatal Intensive Care Units on Infant and Parent Outcomes: A Multicentre, Multinational, Cluster-Randomised Controlled Trial. *The Lancet Child and Adolescent Health*, 2(4): 245–54.

Orsi, K C, Avena, M J, Lurdes de Cacia Pradella-Hallinan, M, da Luz Gonçalves Pedreira, M, Tsunemi, M H, Machado Avelar, A F and Pinheiro, E M (2017) Effects of Handling and Environment on Preterm Newborns Sleeping in Incubators. *Journal of Obstetric, Gynecologic & Neonatal Nursing*, 46(2): 238–47.

Perry, M, Tan, Z, Chen, J, Weidig, T, Xu, W and Cong, XS (2018) Neonatal Pain: Perceptions and Current Practice. *Critical Care Nursing Clinics of North America*, 30(4): 549–61.

Petty, J and van den Hoogen, A (2022) Brain Development, Promoting Sleep and Well-Being in the Context of Neonatal Developmental Care. In Petty,

J, Jones, T, van den Hoogen, A, Walker, K and Kenner, C (eds) *Neonatal Nursing: A Global Perspective* (pp 135–50). Cham: Springer.

Pineda, R G, Neil, J, Dierker, D, Smyser, C D, Wallendorf, M and Kidokoro, H (2014) Alterations in Brain Structure and Neurodevelopmental Outcome in Preterm Infants Hospitalized in Different Neonatal Intensive Care Unit Environments. *Journal of Pediatrics*, 164(1): 52–60.

Séassau, A, Munos, P, Gire, C, Tosello, B and Carchon, I (2023) Neonatal Care Unit Interventions on Preterm Development. *Children*, 10(6): 999.

Siva, N, Nayak, B S, Lewis, L E S, Velayudhan, B, Phagdol, T, Sathish, Y and Noronha, J A (2023) Involvement of Mothers in High-Risk Neonatal Care: A Capacity Building Program for Neonatal Nurses. *Journal of Neonatal Nursing*, 29(1): 91–6.

Williams, K G, Patel, K T, Stausmire, J M, Bridges, C, Mathis, M W and Barkin, J L (2018) The Neonatal Intensive Care Unit: Environmental Stressors and Supports. *International Journal of Environmental Research and Public Health*, 15(1): 60.

Zores, C, Dufour, A, Pebayle, T, Dahan, I, Astruc, D and Kuhn, P (2018) Observational Study Found That Even Small Variations in Light Can Wake Up Very Preterm Infants in a Neonatal Intensive Care Unit. *Acta Paediatrica*, 107(7): 1191–7.

10 Assessment and screening within the clinical neonatal setting

Julia Petty

INTRODUCTION

As seen in Chapter 4, assessment is an essential skill which forms the basis of any decision and subsequent care intervention. Within the neonatal clinical setting, it is an integral and vital component of stabilisation at birth and subsequent clinical care of a neonate thereafter. This chapter focuses on various clinical assessment guides (Figures 10.1 to 10.2; Tables 10.1 to 10.9) to support care within the neonatal unit (NNU) and/or hospital setting.

Chapter learning objectives

By the end of this chapter you will:

✓ be able to gain an overview and understanding of the key principles of assessment relating to the neonate who is receiving clinical neonatal care;

✓ be able to explain how small and premature neonates are assessed and screened.

Critical thinking points

- Consider how assessing a hospitalised neonate is different to one that is healthy.

- What are key factors that require attention in the assessment of a neonate within the hospital/neonatal unit setting?

 Assessment of the *healthy* neonate is covered in Chapter 4.

See the web companion for supplementary information for the topics covered throughout this chapter.

ASSESSMENT OF THE COMPROMISED NEONATE AT BIRTH

 Table 10.1 Assessment of the compromised baby at birth

- **Initial assessment:** Are the following criteria satisfactory at birth: response to stimulation, colour, tone, heart rate and breathing, according to the Newborn Life Support (NLS) algorithm (Resuscitation Council UK, 2021). If concerns are raised, the NLS algorithm may then be commenced – see Chapter 11.

- **Cord care at birth:** If requiring intervention for a concern, immediate cord clamping is performed and the cord is cut, leaving a long segment.

- **Ascertain presence of foetal compromise:** Cardiotocography (CTG) monitoring/ blood gas analysis of cord blood, preferably arterial and venous. Monitor data during labour for presence of thick meconium.

- **Pregnancy:** Were there any pregnancy complications? What was the antenatal history or are there any perinatal factors to consider (eg signs of maternal infection)?

- **Labour:** What was the method of delivery? Was it prolonged/difficult/ instrumental? Did the mother receive antenatal steroids during preterm labour?

- **Gestation:** What is the gestation of the neonate? Was this preterm labour? If the neonate is preterm, is this necessitating specific early care?

- **Care after birth:** Care will be determined by the level of care received on admission to the neonatal unit or postnatal ward/transitional care – see Chapter 11.

- Administer vitamin K at birth – see Chapter 5.

Check local guidance

Follow appropriate local or national guidance on specific aspects of care; for example, for advice on identifying and managing jaundice see the National Institute for Health and Care Excellence (NICE) guidelines on jaundice in newborn babies under 28 days and postnatal care. If there are concerns about the baby's growth, see the NICE guideline on faltering growth.

Stop and think

Consider what is causing the neonate to be compromised – for example, hypoxia, infection, shock or prolonged/difficult labour.

A systematic approach to assessment of the compromised neonate after birth

Assessment of the neonate is multi-factorial. To ensure essential elements of assessment are not missed, a systematic approach is needed to guide the healthcare professional through the process using a logical structure/plan. This can be undertaken using a systems-based (or 'top-to-toe') approach (Table 10.2) or 'A to E' assessment (Figure 10.1).

⊞ Table 10.2 Clinical assessment of the neonate in the hospital setting

System	Normal/expected assessment criteria	Assessment criteria indicating compromise and requiring action
Airway and breathing (respiratory)	**Self-ventilating neonate** – effortless breathing which may be periodic, normal rate, bilateral chest movement, mucous membranes pink in colour, quiet chest sounds, no oxygen requirement, oxygen saturations within normal range. **Ventilated neonate** – even, bilateral chest movement, air entry clear and bilateral, no secretions evident, minimum oxygen requirement.	Tachypnoea, nasal flaring, recession, apnoea, oxygen requirement, grunting, cyanosis, abnormal chest sounds, eg stridor/wheeze, oxygen requirement, poor oxygen saturation. Absent or uneven chest movement, excess secretions, absent breath sounds on one or both sides.
Cardiovascular	Adequate mean blood pressure (MBP), capillary refill <3 seconds, urine output at least 1 ml/kg/hour, mucous membranes pink in colour, warm skin, palpable pulses and heart rate within normal limits.	MBP below desired limit, pale, cool skin, low/diminishing urine output, capillary refill >3 seconds, weak and thready pulses, tachycardia initially, then bradycardia (late sign).
Developmental/ behavioural and stress	No presence of pain or stress. Neonate is positioned appropriately – flexed, limbs in mid-line, appears comfortable, relaxed and able to sleep for long periods.	Presence of pain or stress cues – tense, continual movements, facial expressions, excessive crying and grimace, changes to vital signs, colour change, apnoea, desaturations.

→

Table 10.2 (cont.)

System	Normal/expected assessment criteria	Assessment criteria indicating compromise and requiring action
Environmental/ thermal control	Normal body temperature (36.6–37.2 degrees Celsius) and appropriate environmental temperature according to age and gestation and birth weight.	Temperature <36.6 or >37.3 – ie thermal instability (or 'thermal stress') is present.
Fluid status and balance	Adequate systemic perfusion and urine output (see above), normal/palpable fontanelles, palpable peripheral pulses, good skin turgor, normal sodium level, specific gravity of urine 1.010–1.020, weight gain appropriate for age, equal fluid balance (in and out).	Poor systemic perfusion and low urine output (<1 ml/kg/hour) (see above) or polyuria, sunken or bulging fontanelles, dry skin, fast and thready pulses, high or low specific gravity, large increases or decreases in weight, large positive or negative fluid balance.
Gastro-intestinal and nutritional status	Soft, non-tender abdomen, bowel sounds, nil/minimal aspirate from stomach, which is clear and formed of mucous, bowels open and normal stool, no vomiting, tolerance of feeds if applicable.	Distended, tender, hard abdomen, no bowel sounds or bowel actions, stool bloody/too loose/green/ large and/or increasing stomach aspirates, bile aspirates, vomiting, failure to tolerate feeds.
The 3 Hs (metabolic adaptation)	Able to maintain adequate oxygenation, body temperature and blood glucose. Oxygenation and body temperature – see above, blood glucose >2.5 mmol in first few hours, then 4–6 mmol thereafter.	Failure of normal metabolic adaptation leading to the 3 Hs – hypoxia, hypothermia and hypoglycaemia (<2.5 mmol/L). Hyperglycaemia >8 mmol/L.
Immunological	Signs of infection are not evident.	Signs of infection – eg respiratory distress, colour change, low oxygen saturation, increasing oxygen requirement, changes in vital signs, apnoea.

System	Normal/expected assessment criteria	Assessment criteria indicating compromise and requiring action
Jaundice (hepatic)	Physiological jaundice due to liver immaturity is common: observe clinical jaundice/yellow colouring in sclera of eyes. Serum or transcutaneous bilirubin below treatment threshold.	Jaundice that exceeds threshold bilirubin level requiring treatment or *pathological jaundice* – early onset and due to a disease process.
Muscular–skeletal	Presence of well-toned and flexed posture with spontaneous movements.	Abnormal posture and tone, eg hypo or hypertonia.
Neurological and sensory	Response to stimuli is present. Neonate is alert, wakes for and can feed. Normal/present reflexes are exhibited according to gestation/age.	Unresponsive or less responsive to stimuli, excessive wakefulness or poor levels of consciousness – as above, changes in behaviour. Presence of convulsions.
Skin and general appearance	Normal skin for gestation, eg frail and red in the preterm and well formed in term, pink mucous membranes, no excoriation, no signs of jaundice, umbilical area clean, IV sites healthy.	Broken, excoriated skin, rashes, and tissued IV sites or suspected, clinically jaundiced, blue mucous membranes.

(Adapted from Petty, 2011; Lomax, 2021)

 The focus of the above guide is physical assessment. Family adjustment to admission to a neonatal unit along with assessment of emotional needs is covered in Chapter 12.

 Stop and think

A systematic approach to assessment, particularly using the A to E method (UK Resuscitation Council, 2018), should always follow a logical order, with reassessment before moving on to each subsequent stage.

A – AIRWAY

Patency
Breath sounds

B – BREATHING

Respiratory rate
Chest wall movement
Chest percussion
Lung auscultation
Pulse oximetry

C – CIRCULATION

Colour of mouth mucosa, sweating
Capillary refill time
Palpate pulse rate
Heart auscultation
Blood pressure
Electrocardiography monitoring

D – DISABILITY

Level of consciousness – AVPU: Alert
/Voice responsive/Pain
responsive/Unresponsive
Limb movements
Pupillary light reflexes
Blood glucose

E – EXPOSURE

Assess skin
Temperature

Figure 10.1 'A to E' (ABCDE) assessment

Adapted from Petty (2018) and UK Resuscitation Council (2018, 2021)

TAKING OBSERVATIONS IN THE CLINICAL SETTING

Taking observations of key vital signs is a fundamental nursing skill. It is important that norms are understood as specific to the neonate so that any deviation from this is understood and identified. Tables 10.3 and 10.4, respectively, outline the methods of taking vital signs in the clinical setting and the parameters outside the expected ranges, along with the principles of setting appropriate alarm limits.

⊞ Table 10.3 Taking vital signs in the neonatal unit/clinical setting

Interval	Continuous
Body temperature	
Up to one month old: axilla by digital thermometer.	Via a probe on the abdomen or in the axilla.
Over one month old: axilla by chemical thermometer, 3 minutes, dots against the neonate's trunk and read 10 seconds after removal, OR axilla by digital (as above), OR tympanic thermometer placed in ear canal (NICE, 2013; RCN, 2017).	Continuous readings then influence the incubator or overhead heater setting by being manually changed or by a servo control mechanism. Via a probe on the foot allows peripheral temperature to be observed to consider the core–toe temperature gap.
Heart rate	
Apex: place bell of stethoscope on the apex area – usually to the left of the sternum, between the nipples. Record beats/minute.	Electrocardiograph (ECG). Ensure good sinus rhythm is visible on the monitor.
Pulse	
The brachial or femoral pulse can be palpated in the neonate (under one year of age).	Continuous pulse can be monitored via a pulse oximeter (see below).
Blood pressure	
Non-invasive (cuff) – ensure the cuff covers two-thirds of the upper arm or lower leg. Straighten the limb and keep it still during reading. Either use 'manual' or set the monitor to 'automatic' to be taken at regular intervals	Invasive (arterial) blood pressure – ensure the set-up has been calibrated (zeroed) and the transducer is at the level of heart. Ensure a good trace and optimise. Record hourly.
Respiratory rate	
Observe the chest and count/record breaths per minute. Look for even chest movement, bilateral, ease of breathing.	ECG leads will read a continuous respiratory trace – this should also be checked manually at intervals.

Table 10.3 (cont.)

Interval	Continuous
Oxygen saturation	
Continuous only: a saturation probe attached to a pulse oximeter is placed around a pulsatile area (eg foot, hand, wrist) and the O_2 saturation (SpO_2) and pulse are continuously measured.	
Transcutaneous oxygen	
Continuous only: a probe is calibrated every two to four hours and then placed on a flat surface of the skin – eg chest.	
End tidal carbon dioxide (CO_2)	
Continuous only: CO_2 in exhaled breath is measured at the end of expiration by chemical reaction (calorimetry) or by measuring molecules providing a numerical value (capnometer).	
Capillary refill time (CRT)	
Blanch skin for five seconds and count how many seconds it takes for colour (perfusion) to return.	
Urine output	
Divide urine (ml) passed in each time period by the weight and by the number of hours.	

For *'normal'* ranges and parameters for vital signs, refer to Chapter 4, Table 4.4.

 Check local guidance

Check local guidance on actual devices used for taking vital signs and device/company guidelines.

 Stop and think

All vital signs should be recorded clearly and accurately every hour if a neonate is on continuous monitoring or at intervals, varying from two to four hours. After continuous monitoring has ceased, frequency of vital sign taking and recording generally depends on the individual patient and is agreed accordingly (Royal College of Nursing (RCN), 2017).

Table 10.4 An information guide to abnormal vital signs in a compromised neonate

Vital sign	Normal and abnormal values	Setting limits (upper and lower)
Temperature	**NORMAL**	
	• Central (axilla): 36.6–37.2 degrees Celsius (°C)	Upper limit: 37.5–37.8°C
	• Abdominal (probe): 36.6–37.2°C (preterm)	Lower limit: 36°C
	• Abdominal probe: 35.5–36.5°C (term)	
	• Peripheral (foot): 34.6–36.2°C	
	• Core–toe temperature gap less than 2°C	
	OUTSIDE NORMAL RANGE	
	<36°C = hypothermia	
	>37.8°C = hyperthermia	
Heart rate – beats per minute (bpm)	**NORMAL**	
	• Neonate (preterm): 100–200 bpm (awake)/120–180 bpm (asleep)	100–180 bpm
	• Neonate (term): 100–180 bpm (awake)/80–160 bpm (asleep)	100–160 bpm
	• Infant: 100–160 bpm (awake)/ 75–160 bpm (asleep)	
	OUTSIDE NORMAL RANGE	
	>180–200 bpm = tachycardia	
	<100 bpm = bradycardia	
Respiratory rate – breaths per minute (bpm)	**NORMAL**	
	• Preterm: 40–80 bpm	30–80 bpm
	• Term neonates: 30–70 bpm	30–70 bpm
	• Infants: 30–60 bpm	30–60 bpm
	OUTSIDE NORMAL RANGE	
	>60–80 bpm = tachypnoea	
	<20 bpm = bradypnoea	

→

Table 10.4 (cont.)

Vital sign	Normal and abnormal values	Setting limits (upper and lower)
Blood pressure (mean) (mmHg) **S=systolic** **D=diastolic**	**NORMAL** • birth (12 h, <1 kg): S 39–59/ D 16–36 • birth (12 h, 3 kg): S 50–70/D 24–45 • neonate (96 h): S 60–90/D 20–60 • infant (6 month): S 87–105/ D 53–66 • **Use the gestational age in weeks for acceptable norm of mean blood pressure (MBP)** **OUTSIDE NORMAL RANGE** **<30 mmHg MBP hypotension** **>60–90 (S) & > 30–50 (D) hypertension**	For sick preterm neonate, keep MBP above 30 mmHg For sick term neonate, keep MBP above 40 mmHg
Oxygen saturations	**NORMAL** • Any neonate in air: 90–100% • Term hypoxic neonate: 95–100% • Preterm: SpO_2 should be targeted at 90–94% until the infant reaches 36 weeks postmenstrual age (Sweet et al, 2013) **OUTSIDE NORMAL RANGE** **<90–92% = lower end of acceptable ranges** **<90% and lower = hypoxia**	Term – set lower limit of 90–92% (no need for upper limit) Preterm – set lower and upper alarm limits at 89% and 95% respectively (Sweet et al, 2023) until risk of ROP ceases
Transcutaneous oxygen and CO_2	**NORMAL** • Term – PO_2 – 6.5–12.5 kPa • Preterm – PO_2 – 6.5–10 kPa • Term and preterm – CO_2 – 4–6 kPa **OUTSIDE NORMAL RANGE** **<6.5 PO_2 = hypoxia** **>10.5–12.5 PO_2 = hyperoxia** **>6.5 CO_2 = hypercapnia** **<4 = hypocapnia**	Aim for the same limits as for blood gas values PaO_2 6.5– 10 kPa (preterm)/ 6.5–12 kPa (infant/ child) $PaCO_2$ 4–6 kPa

Check local guidance

Check local guidance on accepted ranges, values and upper/lower limits.

 Stop and think

Setting upper and lower acceptable limits should be done according to the neonate's age, gestation and condition, taking in account factors such as sleep/wake states, activity and stress levels.

ADMISSION TO THE NEONATAL UNIT

A neonate who requires admission to the neonatal unit (NNU) following compromise before, during or after birth will require a full assessment to ascertain baseline values as well as guide subsequent interventions. Table 10.5 outlines a summary guide for NNU admission.

 Table 10.5 Assessment for admission to the neonatal unit

A systematic approach to assessment includes ABC and beyond.

- **A**irway – is it open and patent? What airway support is required?
- **A**ssessment – vital sign observations/monitoring – heart rate, respiratory status, blood pressure, oxygen saturation, blood gas analysis values, blood glucose, admission screen/swabs
- **B**reathing – does the neonate require respiratory support?
- **C**irculation – do they require cardiovascular support?
- **D**rugs – do they require any specific drug therapy?
- **E**nvironment – is the environment prepared? Is it conducive to their needs?
- **F**luid requirement – what fluid regime are they on?
- **G**astro-intestinal/bowels – passed meconium? Abdomen?
- **H** – the 3 Hs (hypoxia, hypoglycaemia or hypothermia)?
- **I**nfection – are there any signs of actual or risk of sepsis?
- **J**aundice – what is the serum bilirubin? Clinical jaundice?

→

Table 10.5 (cont.)

A systematic approach to assessment includes ABC and beyond.

- **K** – vitamin K/Kangaroo care – applicable?
- **L**evel of dependency
- **M**ulti-disciplinary team involvement
- **N**eurological signs
- **O**xygen requirement
- **P**arents
- **Q**uality, risk and safeguarding
- **R**enal/urine
- **S**urgical neonate/skin integrity
- **T**ransfer required.
- **U**mbilical lines and care
- **V**omiting
- **W**eight
- **X**-rays – what are required as part of the assessment above?

 Check local guidance

Check local guidance for specific admission documentation.

 Stop and think

Assessment of a 'baseline' is essential for any neonatal admission as a starting point for any interventions. All admission assessments must be documented.

ASSESSMENT OF THE PRETERM NEONATE

The neonatal unit admits a significant number of preterm neonates for varying levels of care and intervention, many of which are classed as *extremely* preterm. Optimum stabilisation in the early hours of life of these very vulnerable neonates is of utmost importance to optimise their outcome (Wyckoff et al, 2020). There are some specific assessment factors for this group of neonates that require emphasis. Assessment and stabilisation of the preterm neonate at birth is known as the 'Golden Hour' (Harriman et al, 2018). This is outlined in Figure 10.2, which refers to the preterm neonate at less than 32 weeks' gestation. However, a distinction is made between two further sub-sets within this group: those born at less than 28 weeks' gestation and those born *between* 28 weeks and up to 32 weeks. Table 10.6 outlines specific differences relevant to the preterm neonate for clinical assessment and Table 10.7 depicts some key clinical features that can be used to ascertain a neonate's gestational age if this is unknown.

 Stop and think

What happens in the 'Golden Hour' can influence the later outcome of an extremely preterm neonate (Croop et al, 2020).

 Check local guidance

Check local guidance for specific information on care of the preterm neonate.

⊞ Table 10.6 Clinical assessment of the preterm neonate

System	Compared to the term neonate, the key specific features of the preterm neonate are...
Airway and breathing (respiratory)	Immature lung function and surfactant deficiency. Alveoli are more fragile and easily damaged. Underdeveloped respiratory centre leading to a predisposition to apnoea of prematurity.
Cardiovascular	Poor cardiac output due to immaturity of the heart muscle and reduced contractility. Total blood volume is reduced. Higher acceptable heart rate and lower limits for acceptable MBP.
Developmental/ behavioural/ stress	Not able to display the normal behavioural states, posture and movement due to immaturity and lack of muscle development, tone, strength and inability to cry. May exhibit different stress signs or cues.
Environmental/ thermal control	Increased risk of hypothermia due to lack of brown fat and subcutaneous fat, as well as increased surface area to volume ratio. The preterm neonate is more vulnerable to environmental stressors within the extra-uterine environment.

→

Table 10.6 (cont.)

System	Compared to the term neonate, the key specific features of the preterm neonate are...
Fluid status and balance	Immature kidneys which are not able to tolerate large volumes and can easily become overloaded.
Gastro-intestinal and nutrition	Immature gut function and inability to feed orally due to underdeveloped suck–swallow reflexes.
The 3 Hs – metabolic adaptation	Limited glycogen stores and nutritional reserves laid down normally in pregnancy that are more easily exhausted in response to compromise. More prone to the 3 Hs – the preterm neonate is less able to achieve normal metabolic adaptation to extra-uterine life.
Immunological	Prematurity means that neonates will fail to receive the transfer of immunoglobulins across the placenta during the last trimester and will be further immune compromised.
Jaundice (hepatic)	Physiological jaundice is more common due to liver immaturity.
	Lowered threshold for treatment of jaundice.
Muscular-skeletal	Poor muscular tone before 34 weeks' gestation.
Neurological and sensory	Immature germinal matrix (vascular) layer of the brain ventricles under 34 weeks; more prone to intraventricular haemorrhage.
Skin and general appearance	Underdeveloped and poorly waterproofed skin due to lack of keratin.

(Adapted from Kilby et al, 2020; McDonald and Kaiser, 2020)

 Stop and think

The preterm neonate is physiologically immature in all of the above systems, making them particularly vulnerable to the effects of the extra-uterine environment and the impact of neonatal care practices.

At birth

- **All (<32 weeks)**: Assess need for airway management/NLS algorithm, use pulse oximetry to ascertain oxygen requirement.
- **28–32 weeks**: as above *if stable/well*, delay cord clamping, wrap and keep warm, use skin to skin as appropriate.
- **<28 weeks or unstable neonate 28–32 weeks requiring support**: Immediate cord clamping, place neonate in plastic bag (<28–30 weeks) under radiant heater, dry head and put on hat, give airway and breathing support as gently as possible, limit inflation breath pressures.

First hour

- **All (<32 weeks)**: **Key areas:** Stabilisation of airway and breathing, close assessment, sound thermal care, prevention of hypothermia, hypoglycaemia and hypoxia (the 3 Hs).
- **28–32 weeks**: As above. Low threshold for intubation and ventilation. Limit oxygen as much as much as possible; use pulse oximetry and apply limits (See Table 10.4).
- **<28 weeks:** Early surfactant is recommended and the subsequent use of CPAP as tolerated to avoid ventilation. Give oxygen with caution and apply limits as above. Leave in plastic bag and remove when inside humidified incubator (up to 85% humidity). Give gentle handling.

Subsequent care

- **All preterm neonates (< 32 weeks): Key areas**: Aim for early extubation if ventilated, use of CPAP, continued thermal control and humidification, gentle handling and avoidance of stress and pain - no routine suction, minmise environmental influences, early nutrition.
- **For all:** The birth of a preterm neonate has a significant emotional impact on parents. Ensure their needs and anxieties are considered within the 'golden hour' and thereafter.

Figure 10.2 Stabilisation of the preterm neonate: the 'Golden Hour' (Harriman et al, 2018)

⊞ Table 10.7 Assessment of gestational age

SIGN	Extreme preterm		Mid-trimester		Term	Post-term
Skin	Sticky, friable, transparent	Gelatinous, red, translucent	Smooth pink, visible veins	Superficial peeling and/or rash, few veins	Cracking, pale areas, rare veins	Parchment, deep cracking, no vessels	Leathery, cracked, wrinkled
Lanugo hair	None	Sparse	Abundant	Thinning	Bald areas	Mostly bald	n/a
Creases of foot (plantar surface)	No creases	No creases	Faint red marks	Anterior transverse creases only	2/3 creases	Creases over entire sole	n/a
Breast	Not obvious	Barely perceptible	Flat, no bud	Small bud	Raised areola	Full areola	n/a
Eye/ear	Lids fused	Lids open. Ear pinna flat and soft	Curved pinna but soft	Well curved pinna with good recoil	Formed and firm	Thick ear cartilage	n/a
Genitals (male)	Flat smooth scrotum	Scrotum empty	Testes in upper canal	Testes descending, few rugae	Testes down, good rugae	Descended with deep rugae	n/a
Genitals (female)	Clitoris prominent and labia flat	As previous but small labia minora	As previous, growing labia minora	Majora and minora equally prominent	Labia majora large and minora small	Labia majora cover minora	n/a
Posture		Flat and extended	Mild tone present	Some flexion, upper limbs more so than lower	Improved tone and flexion of all limbs	All limbs flexed and toned	

(Adapted from Ballard, 2022)

Stop and think

Knowing the gestational age in weeks of a neonate on admission is important to guide appropriate management.

SCREENING IN THE NEONATAL UNIT

Screening continues to be an important area of healthcare within the clinical setting, as highlighted in Chapter 4. Table 10.8 outlines the specific features of blood spot screening when the neonate is in the NNU. Table 10.9 covers a specific area of screening that is essential for the preterm neonate, relating to retinopathy of prematurity (ROP).

 Table 10.8 Blood spot screening in the neonatal unit

✓ Within five days of birth, a single blood spot is saved for routine sickle cell disease screening to send with the five-to-eight-day test.

✓ On day 5, a full blood spot test is done (unless a blood transfusion has been given).

✓ If a blood transfusion has been given, wait 72 hours before taking the full blood spot test (no later than day 8).

✓ Babies born at less than 32 weeks (less than or equal to 31 weeks + 6 days) require a second blood spot sample (two spots) to be taken, in addition to the day 5 sample, at 28 days of age (counting day of birth as day 0) or day of discharge home, whichever is the sooner.

✓ Record all tests in the Personal Child Health Record or medical notes – indicate date, whether a repeat test and sign.

✓ When multiple blood transfusions and no pre-transfusion blood spot was taken, a repeat test is arranged at three months after the last transfusion.

 Stop and think

When a neonate has had a blood transfusion, either intrauterine or in the newborn period, an interval of at least three clear days is required between the transfusion and the routine blood spot sample (Public Health England, 2021).

Table 10.9 Retinopathy of prematurity

How?	Why?
• **Retinopathy of prematurity (ROP) screening** is undertaken in neonates of less than 1500 g and all neonates of 31 weeks or less.	Done to detect, identify stage and treat ROP as appropriate, as follows...
• First examination is taken at six to seven weeks postnatal age or post-conceptual age of 36 weeks.	**Stage 1: Demarcation line** – thin, relatively flat line separating the vascular and avascular retina.
• Prior to examination cyclopentolate 0.5% and phenylephrine 2.5% eye drops are prescribed and administered prior to the arrival of an ophthalmologist.	**Stage 2: Ridge** – the ridge has height and width extending above the retina.
• Repeat every two weeks or according to individual assessment by the ROP team.	**Stage 3: Proliferation or neovascularisation extends from the ridge into the vitreous.**
• **Location of ROP** – each zone (1–3) is centred around the optic disc as the focal point.	**Stage 4: Partial retinal detachment** – extrafoveal (stage 4a) and foveal (stage 4b) partial retinal detachment.
• **Extent of ROP** – recorded as clock hours.	**Stage 5: Total retinal detachment**

(RCPCH, 2022)

 Check local guidance

In line with national guidance (RCPCH, 2022), also observe local guidance on ROP screening.

 Stop and think

Determination of the stage, location and extent of ROP is used to decide on the need for later treatment by laser or cryotherapy.

 Standard precautions alert

Always apply standard precautions. Wash your hands thoroughly before and after handling neonates during assessment.

See the web companion for a glossary specific to this chapter.

 Check local variations and guidance alert

The space below can be used to record any notes or local variations and practice points specific to your own unit.

REFERENCES

Ballard.com (2022) Ballard Tool for Assessing Gestational Age. [online] Available at: www.ballardscore.com (accessed 5 December 2023).

Croop, S E W, Thoyre, S M, Aliaga, S, McCaffrey, M J and Peter-Wohl, S (2020) The Golden Hour: A Quality Improvement Initiative for Extremely Premature Infants in the Neonatal Intensive Care Unit. *Journal of Perinatology*, 40: 530–9.

Harriman, T L, Carter, B, Dail, R B, Stowell, K E and Zukowsky, K (2018) Golden Hour Protocol for Preterm Infants: A Quality Improvement Project. *Advances in Neonatal Care*, 18(6): 462–70.

Kilby, L, Everett, E, Powis, K and Kyte, E (2020) The Preterm and Low Birthweight Infant. In Boxwell, G, Petty, J and Kaiser, L (eds) *Neonatal Intensive Care Nursing*. 3rd ed (Chapter 3). Abingdon: Routledge.

Lomax, A (2021) *Examination of the Newborn: An Evidence Based Guide*. 3rd ed. Hoboken, NJ: Wiley-Blackwell.

McDonald, L and Kaiser, L (2020) Assessment of the Neonate. In Boxwell, G, Petty, J and Kaiser, L (eds) *Neonatal Intensive Care Nursing*. 3rd ed (Chapter 2). Abingdon: Routledge.

National Institute for Health and Care Excellence (NICE) (2013) Feverish in Under 5s: Assessment and Initial Management. Clinical Guideline [CG160]. [online] Available at: www.nice.org.uk/guidance/cg160 (accessed 5 December 2023).

National Institute for Health and Care Excellence (NICE) (2020) Specialist Neonatal Respiratory Care for Babies Born Preterm: Quality Standard [QS193]. [online] Available at: www.nice.org.uk/guidance/qs193/chapter/Quality-statement-4-Oxygen-saturation (accessed 5 December 2023).

Petty, J (2011) Fact Sheets: Neonatal Biology – An Overview Parts 1, 2 & 3. *Journal of Neonatal Nursing*, 17(2–4): 8–10, 89–91, 128–31.

Petty, J (2018) Principles of Systematic Assessment. In Gormley-Fleming, E and Martin, D (eds) *Children and Young People's Nursing Skills at a Glance* (pp 6–7). Chichester: Wiley-Blackwell.

Public Health England (2021) Newborn Blood Spot Sampling Guidelines: Quick Reference Guide. [online] Available at: www.gov.uk/government/publications/newborn-blood-spot-screening-sampling-guidelines/quick-reference-guide (accessed 5 December 2023).

Royal College of Nursing (RCN) (2017) *Standards for Assessing, Measuring, and Monitoring Vital Signs in Infants, Children, and Young* People. [online] Available at: www.rcn.org.uk/professional-development/publications/pub-005942 (accessed 5 December 2023).

Royal College of Paediatrics and Child Health (RCPCH) (2022) *UK Screening of Retinopathy of Prematurity Guideline.* [online] Available at: www.rcpch.ac.uk/resources/screening-retinopathy-prematurity-rop-clinical-guideline (accessed 5 December 2023).

Sweet, D G, Carnielli, V P, Greisen, G et al (2023) European Consensus Guidelines on the Management of Respiratory Distress Syndrome: 2022 Update. *Neonatology*, 120(1): 3–23.

UK Resuscitation Council (2018) The ABCDE Approach. [online] Available at: www.resus.org.uk/library/abcde-approach (accessed 5 December 2023).

UK Resuscitation Council (2021) *Newborn Resuscitation and Support of Transition of Infants at Birth Guidelines.* [online] Available at: www.resus.org.uk/library/2021-resuscitation-guidelines/newborn-resuscitation-and-support-transition-infants-birth (accessed 5 December 2023).

Wyckoff, M H, Wyllie, J, Aziz, K et al (2020) Neonatal Life Support: 2020 International Consensus on Cardiopulmonary Resuscitation and Emergency Cardiovascular Care Science with Treatment Recommendations. *Circulation*, 142(16): S185–S221.

11 Important practices in the neonatal intensive care unit

Julia Petty

INTRODUCTION

The sickest and most premature neonates often require admission to a high level of 'dependency', including the neonatal intensive care unit (NICU). This chapter covers important principles of care that are relevant to more intensive dependency levels within the neonatal unit setting, namely, resuscitation, ventilation practice, taking blood, cardiovascular care and drug administration (Figures 11.1 to 11.16; Tables 11.1 to 11.12).

Chapter learning objectives

By the end of this chapter you will:

✓ have gained knowledge and insight into a range of practices relevant to caring for the neonate in high dependency and the NICU setting;

✓ be able to understand the challenges and complexities faced by neonates and families in higher-dependency settings.

Critical thinking points

• Consider the different needs of a sick and/or premature infant who requires high dependency and/or admission to the NICU.

• What are the key priorities of care in relation to positive outcomes and to prevent complications by deterioration or iatrogenic risk?

 See Chapter 8 for other fundamental areas of practice in the neonatal unit setting.

See the web companion for supplementary information for the topics covered throughout this chapter.

NEONATAL RESUSCITATION

A standardised and structured approach is necessary for any resuscitation.

Resuscitation at birth

The majority of newborn babies breathe spontaneously within the first few minutes of life and open their airway adequately to ventilate and oxygenate themselves to sustain life after delivery. However, there are times in neonatal care when airway management and resuscitation is required relating to the neonate's condition at birth or thereafter.

 Stop and think

Preparation and checking the Resuscitaire® (if available – Figure 11.1) and/or resuscitation equipment (Figure 11.2) is essential at least daily to ensure readiness for emergency and unexpected events. See the web companion for a full list of necessary resuscitation equipment.

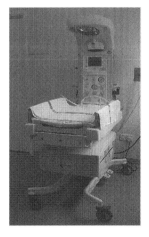

Figure 11.1 Resuscitaire®

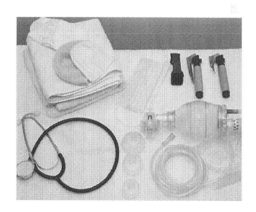

Figure 11.2 Resuscitation equipment

Figure 11.3a depicts the Newborn Life Support (NLS) algorithm (UK Resuscitation Council, 2021) with additional information given in Figure 11.3b. The *order* of interventions is important and reassessment for a response is essential after *each stage* or intervention to move on through the algorithm.

Newborn baby at delivery
Dry the baby (exceptions apply, eg the premature infant to be placed in a plastic bag).
Remove wet towel and cover/keep warm.
Start clock/note time/call for help.

Assess colour, tone, breathing and heart rate

If not breathing
A. Open the airway (neutral position, see Figure 11.4).

If still not breathing
B. Give five inflation breaths using air initially for term babies.
(Add oxygen for premature infant, according to pulse oximetry.)
(2–3 seconds each at pressure 30 cm/H_2O for term OR max 25 cm/H_2O for premature.)

Look for a response
Ask: has the heart rate increased? Is the chest moving?
If no increase in heart rate, look for chest movement.

If no response
Recheck head position, apply jaw thrust.
Repeat inflation breaths, look for a response.
If no increase in heart rate, look for chest movement.

If still no response
Try alternative airway opening manoeuvres.
Repeate inflation breaths, look for a response.
If no increase in heart rate, look for chest movement.

Continue repeating inflation breaths until there is a response

When the chest is moving
Give ventilation breaths at 30 per minute and check the heart rate.

If the heart rate is not detectable or slow (<60 per minute)
CALL FOR HELP
C. Start good quality chest compressions immediately at ratio 3:1.
Either thumbs or two fingers just under the nipple line. Press one third chest depth.

Reassess every 30 seconds
D. Consider venous access and drugs if no increase in heart rate.

If heart rate increases, stop compressions and continue ventilation breaths at 30 per minute

Figure 11.3a Newborn Life Support (NLS) algorithm
(UK Resuscitation Council, 2021)

Normal oxygen saturation (SpO$_2$) readings (via pulse oximetry) at birth

- **Acceptable pre-ductal SpO$_2$ (via right hand):** 2 minutes 65%, 5 minutes 85%, 10 minutes 90%.

Airway opening manoeuvre

- 2-person jaw thrust, one to apply jaw thrust and the other to give manual breaths.
- Inspection of the oropharynx under *direct vision* and *suction only if necessary.*
- Insertion of an airway adjunct under *direct vision.*

Resuscitation drug dosages

- **Adrenaline:** Intravenous (IV) is the preferred route, intra-osseous (IO) is an alternative: 20 micrograms/kg (0.2 ml kg of 1:10,000 adrenaline, 1000 micrograms in 10 ml). Use intra-tracheal route if intubated and no other access available. 100 micrograms/kg (1.0 ml/kg of 1:10,000 adrenaline [1000 micrograms in 10 mL). If tracheal adrenaline is given IV or IO access should still be sought. Subsequent doses every 3–5 minutes if heart rate remains <60/min.
- **Glucose:** In a prolonged resuscitation to reduce likelihood of hypoglycaemia. IV or IO: 250 mg/kg bolus (2.5 ml/kg of 10% glucose solution).
- **Volume replacement:** With suspected blood loss or shock unresponsive to other resuscitative measures. IV or IO: 10 ml/kg of group O Rh-negative blood or isotonic crystalloid.
- **Sodium bicarbonate:** May be considered in a prolonged unresponsive resuscitation to reverse intracardiac acidosis. IV or IO: 1–2 mmol/kg sodium bicarbonate (2–4 ml/kg of 4.2% solution) by slow IV injection.

Figure 11.3b Newborn Life Support (NLS)

(Resuscitation Council, 2021)

 Stop and think

Remember ABCD in that order (Airway, Breathing, Circulation, Drugs). Most newborns require A and B only, due to the primary reason for resuscitation in this age group. Only a few require C and D.

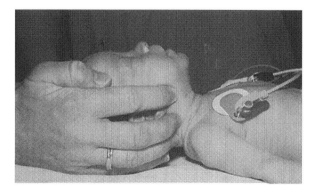

Figure 11.4 The neutral position

(Reproduced with the kind permission of Resuscitation Council UK)

Resuscitation in the neonatal unit

The NLS algorithm applies to all neonates within a hospital setting until they are discharged home, when the paediatric guidelines become applicable. Resuscitation may be required when an infant in the neonatal or postnatal unit suddenly deteriorates (Figure 11.5).

Move the neonate to a Resuscitaire® *or* flat, firm surface.

Call for help.
Access emergency trolley/equipment.
Note time.

Assess: Airway
Neutral position, suction mouth and/or nose *if indicated.*

Assess: Breathing
Use 'T-piece' inflation or bag-valve mask (self-inflating bag). Five breaths lasting 2–3 seconds looking for chest movement and/or increase in heart rate.

If no chest movement, reposition airway, provide jaw thrust.

Listen for heart rate and chest movement. If chest is moving and heart rate has increased provide ventilation breaths to support breathing.

If chest is moving and heart rate is less than 60
Assess: Circulation
Perform cardiac compressions at a ratio of 3:1 (if newborn) OR 15:2 if paediatric guidelines are followed.

Reassess every 30 seconds.
If heart rate remains <30, consider IV access and drugs.

If the infant is intubated/ventilated, listen to air entry with a stethoscope.

CONSIDER THE FOLLOWING: DOPES
> **D**isplacement of endotracheal tube (ETT)?
> **O**bstruction of ETT?
> **P**neumothorax? Pulmonary haemorrhage?
> **E**quipment malfunction? Are there any leaks or equipment faults?
> **S**tiff lungs? The lungs may become less compliant due to collapse, lung oedema or abdominal distension.

Figure 11.5 ABC: resuscitation in the neonatal unit

 Stop and think

The same standard approach highlighted above for the newborn NLS algorithm applies to any neonate that requires resuscitation in all settings, again with the main focus on airway and breathing.

VENTILATION IN THE NEONATAL UNIT

A healthy neonate with an open airway will be able to breathe spontaneously without problems. However, in neonatal care, respiratory management to support a neonate's breathing is often necessary. Non-invasive means of support are always preferable to avoid potential long-term damage to lungs from mechanical ventilation. The aim is to wean any support as soon as possible and for the neonate to breathe on their own. The next section covers ventilation strategies, starting with continuous positive airway pressure (CPAP) and then considering more invasive means of positive pressure ventilation (Figures 11.6 to 11.14, Tables 11.1 to 11.4).

Continuous positive airway pressure (CPAP)

CPAP is administered non-invasively by a flow driver (shown in Figure 11.6), via two short nasal prongs (Figure 11.7) or via a mask over both nostrils. The flow driver offers a selection of modes to avoid the need for intubation/reintubation and to assist in weaning the neonate off mechanical ventilation. One CPAP level can be given or two (biphasic).

⊞ Table 11.1 Biphasic positive airway pressure (BiPAP)

Knowledge point	Practice implication
Infant flow SIPAP© provides bi-level nasal CPAP.	A baseline pressure is set as well as extra pulses or 'sighs' (brief periods of increased pressure).
Baseline pressure, a set flow of 8–10 litres/minute (on the 'low pressure' flow dial), is set to obtain pressure.	8–10 litres/minute should give a pressure of 4–6 cm/water, provided that there is an adequate seal at the nostrils. Altering the flow will affect the pressure given.
For the additional pressure, set this using the second 'high pressure' flow dial – set at 2 litres/minute.	The pulses or 'sighs' of increased pressure above the baseline CPAP pressure may be timed or 'triggered' by neonate's own inspiratory efforts.
A special 'flip' mechanism in the connection to the nose supports the neonate's breathing throughout both inspiration and expiration.	The continuous gas flow provides a residual and stable gas CPAP pressure delivery throughout the respiratory cycle. When expiration stops, the flow instantly flips back to the inspiratory position.
Modes	
CPAP	One level of pressure. It can be given with or without an 'apnoea' transducer placed onto the abdomen.
Biphasic timed	A baseline pressure is set, and the extra pressure supported 'sighs' are delivered according to a set 'rate' and inspiratory time.
Biphasic trigger	As above but the extra pressure sighs are not timed but triggered by the neonate initiating a breath.
Biphasic + apnoea	As for *biphasic timed* but there is additional apnoea monitoring, and an alarm will sound if the neonate does not breathe within the apnoea interval (as for CPAP and apnoea above).

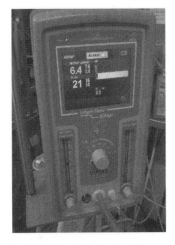

↗ Figure 11.6 CPAP infant flow driver

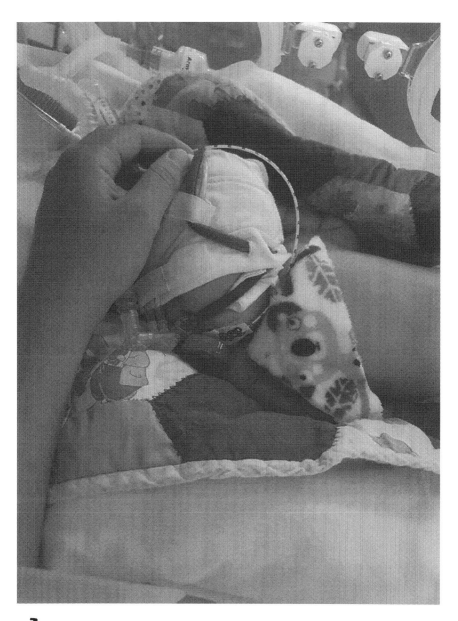

 Figure 11.7 Premature neonate receiving nasal CPAP

👋 *Stop and think*

CPAP should always be considered before more invasive models of intubation and full ventilation in line with a protective lung strategy.

Table 11.2 Nursing care of the neonate on CPAP: specific practice points

A balance is necessary between an adequate seal at the nose to maintain pressure **and prevention of nasal trauma.** This can be done by:

- ensuring the nasal prongs/mask/bonnet are sized correctly according to guidelines;
- ensuring the bonnet to nose strapping provides secure fixation but is not too tight;
- positioning the neonate and the tubing appropriately so that it is well supported;
- regularly checking for nasal trauma;
- assessing the neonate for any discomfort and providing a measure to settle and console;
- continuous monitoring of vital signs including oxygen monitoring;
- humidification of CPAP gases, which is essential;
- assessing the need the oral/nasal suction, only if required;
- giving mouth care regularly due to potential dryness from gases;
- continuing feeding while on CPAP if applicable – observe for abdominal distention; nasogastric tube should be in situ and left on free drainage if neonate is not fed OR to be aspirated before each feed and any excess gas removed.

(Petty, 2013)

 Check local guidance

Check local guidance on setting up CPAP/BiPAP, weaning pressures and specific care.

POSITIVE PRESSURE VENTILATION

Sometimes referred to as intermittent positive pressure ventilation (IPPV), mechanical or artificial ventilation, this term applies to the delivery of positive pressure to a neonate via an endotracheal tube (Figure 11.8) and a ventilator (Figure 11.9) according to set parameters (Figure 11.10). Table 11.3 provides a summary of current ventilation recommendations based on current evidence and Table 11.4 explains ventilation terminology.

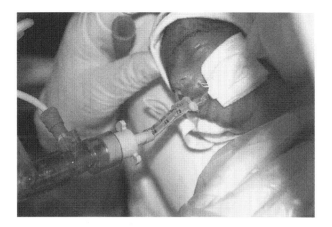

Figure 11.8 Intubated premature neonate receiving mechanical ventilation

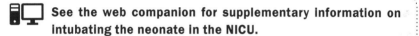

See the web companion for supplementary information on intubating the neonate in the NICU.

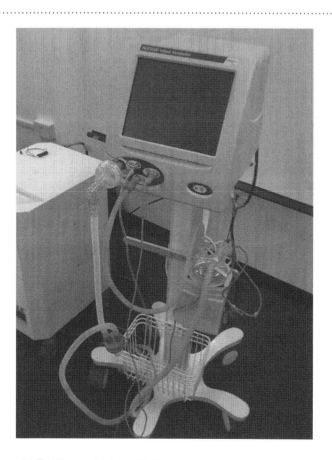

Figure 11.9 Mechanical ventilator

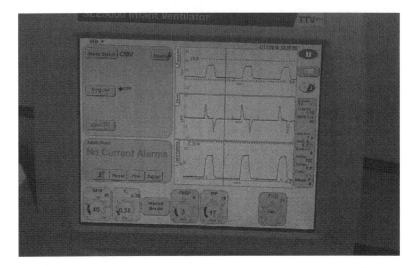

↗ Figure 11.10 Ventilator screen showing parameters set and measured graphic waveforms

❓ Table 11.3 A guide to neonatal respiratory practice (Sweet et al, 2023)

Prenatal care

- Mothers at high risk of preterm birth <28–30 weeks of gestation should be transferred to expert perinatal centres.
- In some women (singleton pregnancy, short cervix in mid-pregnancy, previous preterm birth), vaginal progesterone may be used to increase gestational age at delivery and reduce perinatal mortality and morbidity.
- In women with symptoms of preterm labour, cervical length and accurate biomarker measurements should be considered to prevent unnecessary use of tocolytic drugs and/or antenatal steroids.
- A single course of prenatal corticosteroids should be offered to women at risk of preterm delivery, up to 34 weeks of gestation, ideally at least 24 h before birth.
- A single repeat course of steroids may be given in threatened preterm birth before 32 weeks of gestation if the first course was administered at least one to two weeks earlier.
- Magnesium sulphate ($MgSO_4$) should be administered to women with imminent delivery before 32 weeks of gestation.
- Short-term use of tocolytic drugs in very preterm pregnancies may allow completion of a course of prenatal corticosteroids and/or in utero transfer to a perinatal centre.

Delivery room stabilisation

- If clinical condition allows, defer clamping the umbilical cord for at least 60 seconds. Only when delayed cord clamping (DCC) is not feasible, consider umbilical cord milking in infants with gestational age >28 weeks.

- T-piece devices should be used rather than a bag and mask and spontaneously breathing preterm infants should be stabilised using CPAP. If apnoeic or bradycardic, give ventilation breaths. Start with CPAP pressure at least 6 cm H_2O and peak inspiratory pressures 20–25 cm H_2O.

- Oxygen for resuscitation should be controlled using a blender using an initial FiO_2 of 0.30 for infants <28 weeks of gestation and 0.21–0.30 for those 28–31 weeks and 0.21 for 32 weeks of gestation and above. Adjustments should be guided by pulse oximetry. SpO_2 of 80% or more (and heart rate >100 bpm) should be achieved within five minutes.

- Intubation should be reserved for babies not responding to positive pressure ventilation via face mask or nasal prongs.

- Plastic bags or occlusive wrapping under radiant warmers and humidified gas should be used during stabilisation for babies <32 weeks of gestation to reduce the risk of hypothermia. Hyperthermia should also be avoided.

Surfactant therapy

- If a preterm baby <30 weeks of gestation requires intubation for stabilisation, give an animal-derived surfactant.

- Less-invasive surfactant administration (LISA) is the preferred method of surfactant administration for spontaneously breathing babies on CPAP.

- Laryngeal mask surfactant may be used for more mature infants >1.0 kg.

- Rescue surfactant should be given early in the course of respiratory distress syndrome (RDS).

- A second and occasionally a third dose of surfactant should be given if there is a persistent high oxygen requirement and other problems have been excluded.

Oxygen monitoring

In preterm babies receiving oxygen, the saturation target should be between 90 and 94% with alarm limits set to 89% and 95%.

Protocols for screening and treating preterm babies for retinopathy of prematurity (ROP) should be in place.

Non-invasive ventilation (NIV)

- CPAP or synchronised nasal intermittent positive pressure ventilation ((s)NIPPV) should be started from birth in all babies at risk of RDS, such as those <30 weeks of gestation who do not need intubation for stabilisation.

- NIV with early rescue surfactant by the LISA technique is considered optimal management.

- CPAP interface should be short binasal prongs or mask with a starting pressure of about 6–8 cm H_2O.

- BiPAP devices confer no advantage over CPAP alone. However, synchronised NIPPV, if delivered through a ventilator, can reduce need for ventilation or need for re-ventilation following extubation and may reduce BPD.

- High flow nasal cannula (HFNC) oxygen can be used as an alternative to CPAP for some babies, with the advantage of less nasal trauma, provided that centres have access to CPAP or NIPPV for those failing this mode.

$\rightarrow$

Table 11.3 (cont.)

Mechanical ventilation (MV) strategies

- MV should be used in babies with RDS when other methods of respiratory support have failed. Duration of MV should be minimised.

- Lung-protective modes such as VTV or high-frequency oscillation ventilation should be the first choice for babies with RDS who require MV.

- When weaning from MV, it is reasonable to tolerate a modest degree of hypercarbia, provided the pH remains above 7.22 (B2). Avoid pCO_2 <4.7 kPa (35 mm Hg) when on MV to reduce brain injury.

- INO in preterm babies should be limited to a therapeutic trial for those in whom there is documented pulmonary hypertension with severe respiratory distress and stopped if there is no response.

- Caffeine (20 mg/kg loading, 5–10 mg/kg maintenance) should be used to facilitate weaning from MV. Early caffeine can be considered for babies at high risk of needing MV such as preterm babies on NIV.

- A short tapering course of low-dose dexamethasone should be considered to facilitate extubation in babies who remain on MV after one to two weeks.

- Opioids should be used selectively when indicated by clinical judgement and evaluation of pain indicators. The routine use of morphine or midazolam infusions in ventilated preterm infants is not recommended.

(Recommendations from Sweet et al, 2023; NICE, 2019)

 Stop and think

Selecting the right mode of ventilation is determined by the neonate's condition, state of the lungs and response to existing interventions. What is right for one neonate may not necessarily suit another.

Table 11.4 Ventilation parameters, useful formulas and definitions

Parameter	Definition
Fraction of inspired oxygen (FiO$_2$)	How much oxygen is delivered – expressed as a fraction of 1. Can also be expressed as a percentage.
Mean airway pressure (MAP)	The total pressure (in cm H_2O) within the lungs throughout the respiratory cycle as determined by PIP, PEEP, Ti and Te. Along with FiO$_2$, this influences oxygenation. $$\frac{Rate \times Ti \times (PIP + PEEP) + PEEP - MAP}{60}$$ (Chang, 2011)

Parameter	Definition
Tidal volume (Vt)	The volume of gas entering the lungs in one breath. Expressed in millilitres (ml). Recommended tidal volume (Vt) = 4–6 ml/kg.
Minute volume (Vmin)	The volume of gas entering the lungs over one minute expressed as litres/minute. Minute volume is tidal volume multiplied by the rate and affects CO_2 elimination. Vmin = Vt × rate.
Ventilator parameters (Conventional)	
Rate	The number of breaths delivered in a minute – as breaths per minute (bpm).
Peak inspiratory pressure (PIP)	Peak pressure reached at the end of inspiration (cm H_2O).
Positive end expiratory pressure (PEEP)	End pressure reached at the end of expiration (cm H_2O).
Inspiratory time (Ti)	The inspiratory time of one respiratory cycle expressed in seconds. Range is 0.35–0.4 seconds.
Expiratory time (Te)	The expiratory time of one respiratory cycle expressed in seconds. With a constant or pre-determined Ti, the Te will vary depending on the required rate.
I:E ratio	The ratio of inspiration to expiration time. Te should be longer than Ti.
Flow	The flow of gas delivered. Expressed as litres per minute (L/min).
Trigger threshold	The sensitivity of the ventilator and flow sensor to detect the neonate's breaths and trigger the ventilator.
Leak	Flow that is lost from the respiratory circuit. Measured as the difference between inspiratory and expiratory flow.
Parameters in high-frequency oscillation ventilation (HFOV)	
MAP	As above – controls oxygenation along with FiO_2.
Frequency	Measured in Hertz (Hz) – 60 oscillations in 1 Hz. Set as 8–10 Hz.

→

Table 11.4 (cont.)

Parameter	Definition	
Amplitude	The variation round the MAP. Also known as delta P or power and affects chest 'wiggle'. Controls CO_2 elimination. Set according to extent of chest wiggle/ bounce and blood gas analysis.	
Other ventilation terms		
Functional residual capacity (FRC)	The volume of gas present in the lung alveoli at the end of passive expiration.	FRC is reduced in conditions such as respiratory distress syndrome (RDS) where there is poor lung compliance.
Compliance	The elasticity of the respiratory system.	Compliance = volume/ pressure. The volume/pressure loop displayed represents the relationship graphically.
Resistance	The capability of the airways and endotracheal tube to oppose airflow. Expressed as the change in pressure per unit change in flow.	Resistance = pressure/flow. Again, this is displayed graphically on some ventilators.

(Adapted from Petty, 2013)

 Check local guidance

Check local guidance and model of ventilator for terminology used.

MAKING CHANGES TO VENTILATION

Ventilation should be delivered in a dynamic fashion and should continually be reviewed with the aim to reduce requirements as soon as possible. Ventilation should be delivered in a dynamic fashion and should continually be reviewed with the aim to reduce requirements as soon as possible. When changing ventilation, it is important to understand general principles, as follows.

Manipulating oxygenation: MAP controls oxygenation. So oxygenation can be influenced by changing any of the variables that alter MAP (PIP, PEEP, Ti and Te).

Manipulating CO_2 elimination: minute volume (Vmin) controls CO_2 elimination. CO_2 levels will be influenced by any changing measure which affects Vmin (ie manipulating the rate, Vt or both will alter the Vmin; remember: Vmin = Vt x rate).

Stop and think

The intention to wean along with any weaning strategy should be in place as soon as a neonate is started on any means of ventilation support, being mindful of limiting pressure, volume and oxygen.

 See the web companion for supplementary information on changing and weaning ventilation.

Other ventilation care practices

There are many areas to consider when caring for a neonate on artificial ventilation by any means, covered in brief in Figures 11.11 to 11.14. Ventilation requires gases delivered to the lungs to be warmed and humidified to prevent adverse consequences for the vulnerable airway such as drying, thickening and poor clearance of secretions and increased risk of infection. In addition, to ventilate effectively, the endotracheal tube (ETT) must remain patent and clear of secretions that may interfere with the adequacy of ventilation. Care and checking of equipment are also necessary, including the ventilator flow sensor. There are times when other more advanced interventions are required in the very sick neonate such as chest drain insertion and the use of inhaled nitric oxide.

 See the web companion for further detail and supplementary information on these ventilation practices.

Airway humidification

Any artificial ventilation mode delivering gas to the airway and lungs must deliver warmed gases via a humidifier to avoid any potential damage (Figure 11.11).

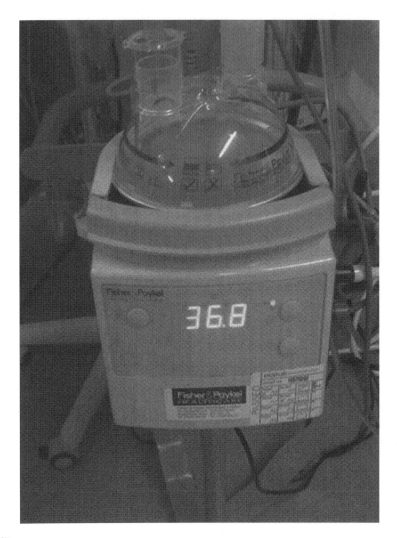

Figure 11.11 Humidifier

Suctioning the airway

Suctioning the airway is performed to maintain its patency by safe removal of secretions. In neonatal practice, suctioning can be undertaken via the nasopharyngeal (NP), oropharyngeal (OP) or endotracheal tube (ETT) route.

○   **NP/OP suctioning.** At birth it may be necessary to clear thick meconium, blood or vernix (rarely) to ensure an open airway when breathing is being established. For the non-ventilated neonate in NICU, suction may be required to clear copious, thick oral or nasal secretions during a chest infection or when on CPAP.

○ **Endotracheal tube (ETT) suctioning.** Suctioning the ETT in the ventilated neonate should be performed only when indicated, based on clinical assessment, to prevent a blocked tube. A closed suction system is preferable to avoid disconnection from the ventilator (Figure 11.12).

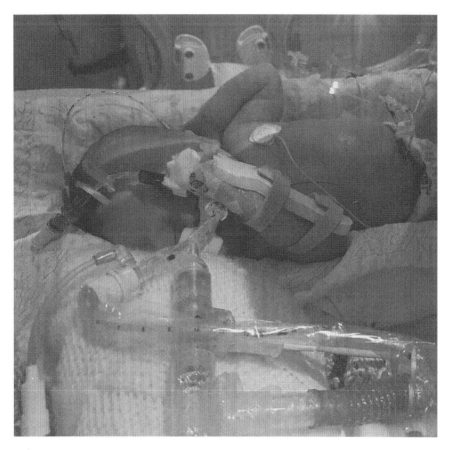

Figure 11.12 Ventilated infant in NICU with a closed suction unit (in foreground)

Calibration of flow sensor

This should be done at the start of each shift to ensure accurate measurements of flow pressure and volume as displayed on the ventilator screen.

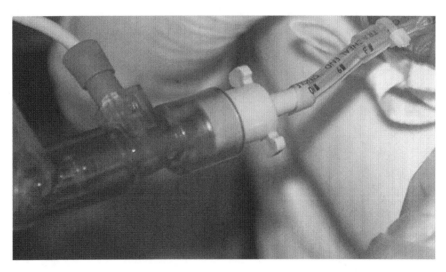

Figure 11.13 Ventilator flow sensor

Chest drain care

Chest drain insertion is undertaken to remove unwanted air in the presence of an air leak such as a pneumothorax or to drain fluid in the case of a pleural effusion. Diagnosis of an air leak is carried out using either a cold light (chest transillumination) or definitively by chest X-ray. Figure 11.14 shows a diagram of a chest drain set-up on an infant.

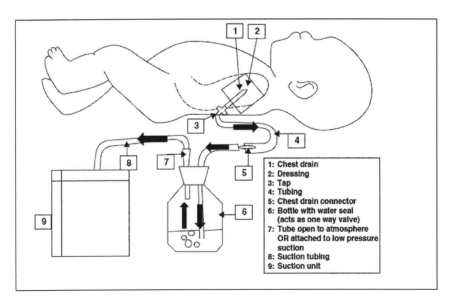

Figure 11.14 Chest drain set-up

Inhaled nitric oxide

Inhaled nitric oxide (iNO) therapy can be considered medically necessary for hypoxic respiratory failure associated with evidence of persistent pulmonary hypertension of the newborn (PPHN) to improve the oxygenation index. Evidence suggests that inhalation of nitric oxide of 20 parts per million (ppm) has been found to be effective in most neonates and such a dose is the standard starting dose followed by titration. iNO is generally administered over a maximum period of five days.

 Standard precautions alert

Care must be taken during suction not to introduce infection by using an aseptic non-touch technique and sterile gloves. Ensure that each catheter used is inserted once only (single use) and then discarded.

The chest drain procedure is undertaken using a strict aseptic technique and there are key nursing responsibilities before, during and after the procedure to maintain optimum safety and comfort of the neonate.

BLOOD VALUES IN NEONATAL CARE

Sampling blood by varying means for analysis, screening and/or diagnosis is a very common practice in neonatal care. It is therefore important to understand normal blood parameters (Table 11.5). Understanding blood values specific to the neonatal group is important as there are some physiological differences in this group compared to the older child and adult.

Normal blood values

Table 11.5 outlines normal values and ranges for the common blood tests taken in the neonatal unit.

 Stop and think

As for vital signs assessment, the frequency of taking blood for the various tests that may be necessary should be decided on an individual basis.

Table 11.5 Blood values in the neonate

Electrolytes	Normal values
Alkaline phosphatase (0–2 years)	100–350 iu
Ammonia	<40–50 micromols/L
Amylase	8–85 iu
Aspartate transaminase (AST)	15–45 u/L
Bicarbonate	18–25 mmol/L
Bilirubin (total)	2–24 micromol/L
Bilirubin (conjugated)	up to 4 micromol/L
Calcium (ionised)	1.2–1.3 mmol/L
Calcium (total)	2.1–2.6 mmol/L
Chloride	9–110 mmol
Creatinine	60–120 micromol/L
Glucose	3.6–5.4 mmol/L
Insulin	<15 mu/L
Iron	9–27 micromol/L
Lactate (venous)	1–1.8 mmol/L
Magnesium	0.7–1 mmol/L
Phosphate	1.3–2.1 mmol/L
Potassium	3.5–5.5 mmol/L
Protein (total)	57–80 g/L
Albumin	33–47 g/L
Globulin	17–38 g/L
Plasma osmolarity	270–295 mmol/kg
Sodium	135–145 mmol/L
Urea	1.0–8.5 mmol/L

Full blood count values

	Cord blood	24 hours	1 week
Term infants			
Mean Hb (g/dL)	16.8	18.4	17
Range WBC (×10/9/L)	10–26	14–31	6–15
Platelets (×10/9/L)		150–400	
Preterm infants			
Mean Hb (g/dL)	14.5		
Range WBC (×10/9/L)	5–19	5–21	6–18
Platelets (×10/9/L)		100–350	

	28 wks	34 wks	Term	Day 1	Day 3	Day 7	Day 14
Hb	14.5	15	16.8	18.4	17.8	17	16.8
HCT %	45	47	53	58	55	54	52

General ranges for year 1 of life

Haematocrit (HCT) or also called PCV – packed cell volume	0.35–0.45 (35–45%)
Haemoglobin	9–14.5 g/dL
Platelets	150–400 ×10/L
White cells	6–18
Neutrophils	2–8.5
Lymphocytes	1–5.4
Monocytes	0.2–0.8

Clotting values

TERM

Test (seconds)	Day 1	Day 5	Day 30	Adult
Prothrombin time (PT)	13	12.4	11.8	12.4
Partial thromboplastin time (PTT)	42.9	42.6	40.4	33.5
Fibrinogen (g/L)	2.83	3.12	2.7	2.78

(NB Values are averages and variations around the mean exist by + or minus 1–1.5 seconds)

→

Table 11.5 (cont.)

PRETERM

Test (seconds)	Day 1	Day 5	Day 30	Adult
Prothrombin time (PT)	13	12.5	11.8	12.4
Partial thromboplastin time (PTT)	53.6	50.5	44.7	33.5
Fibrinogen (g/L)	2.43	2.8	2.54	2.78

(NB Values are averages and variations around the mean exist by + or minus 1–1.5 seconds)

SUMMARY

Prothrombin time	12–18 seconds
PTT	29–52 seconds
TT	8–12 seconds
Fibrinogen	1–8.4 g/L
Other values	
CRP	<2 mg/L (although a trend is most important)
Lactate	<3–5 mmol/L

(Rennie, 2012)

Blood gas analysis

A vital and common investigation for assessment of the sick or compromised neonate in clinical care is blood gas analysis, which gives valuable information regarding a neonate's respiratory, oxygenation and metabolic status along with the response to changes to management, such as ventilation changes and administration of oxygen and fluids. Table 11.6 and Figure 11.15 outline blood gas analysis and values.

 Stop and think

It should be remembered that exceptions to 'normal', 'textbook' values apply, depending on the individual situation – for example, permissive hypercapnia, compensated values, site of sampling. These must be considered in the interpretation of blood gases.

⊞ Table 11.6 Blood gas values in the neonatal unit

	pH	CO$_2$	O$_2$	Bicarbonate	Base	Lactate
CORD (arterial)	7.25–7.28	48 mmHg 6.5 kPa	27–38 mmHg 3.8–5 kPa	n/a	–4	Normal cord lactate: 1.5–4.5 mmol/L
CORD (venous)	7.28–7.35	35–45 mmHg 5–6 kPa	18–22.5 mmHg 2.4–3 kPa	n/a	–4	
NEONATAL (arterial)	7.35–7.45	35–45 mmHg (38) 4.6–6 kPa	50–90 mmHg 7–12 kPa Term 50–80 mmHg 6.5–10.5 kPa Preterm	22–26 mEq/L Term 20–24 mEq/L Preterm Or 22–26 mmol	+2 to –2	Normal neonatal lactate: <2 mmol/L

FOR 'uncompensated' gas (ie pH is abnormal)

Low pH and high CO$_2$ = respiratory acidosis

Low pH and large base deficit/low bicarbonate = metabolic acidosis

High pH and low CO$_2$ = respiratory alkalosis

High pH and large base excess/high bicarbonate = metabolic alkalosis

Low pH, high CO$_2$ and large base deficit = mixed acidosis

FOR 'compensated' gas (ie pH is normal but other values are out of range)

pH	CO$_2$	Bicarbonate	Problem
Low normal	High	High	Compensated respiratory acidosis
High normal	Low	Low	Compensated respiratory alkalosis
Low normal	Low	Low	Compensated metabolic acidosis
High normal	High	High	Compensated metabolic alkalosis

(Petty, 2013; Arias-Oliveras, 2016)

 Check local guidance

Check local guidance on agreed/acceptable blood gas norms and ranges.

 Stop and think

Consider the following additional notes.

- **Permissive hypercapnia**. Accept different to the normal range outlined previously. To avoid over-ventilating the lungs, keep pH >7.25.

→

- **kPa or mmHg?** Values are expressed in both kPa *and* mmHg for $PaO_2/PaCO_2$ and in mEq/L *and* mmol for bicarbonate to account for differences between countries.

- **Arterial, capillary or venous?** Arterial blood is preferred for the most accurate values. Capillary venous neonatal sampling can be considered for all values (pH, CO_2, base and bicarbonate) *except oxygenation status.*

1: ASSESS pH

Is the pH normal? If not, is it acidotic or alkalotic?

2: ASSESS RESPIRATORY COMPONENT

Is CO_2 within normal range?

3: ASSESS METABOLIC COMPONENT

Is the bicarbonate within normal range and is there a large base deficit or excess?

4: ASSESS IF COMPENSATION HAS OCCURED

ie has the pH normalised but the other values are out of normal range?

5: ASSESS OXYGENATION (PaO$_2$)

A low PaO_2 can contribute to a metabolic acidosis by anaerobic respiration by cells and lactic acidosis accumulation.

Plus
CONSIDER LACTATE LEVELS

6: INTERPRET AND MAKE PLAN OF ACTION

7: EVALUATE/REASSESS

 Figure 11.15 Interpretation of blood gases in the neonatal unit

Stop and think

A systematic approach to working through the different aspects of a blood gas analysis result is useful, always considering the pH *as a priority* and then leading on to working out what has contributed to the change in pH.

Blood sampling from neonates

 Table 11.7 A guide to taking blood tests – some tips and important points

---

What method is appropriate? Heel prick, venepuncture or arterial line sampling?

- If cannulation or arterial line is inserted, take any required blood at the same time.

- If an arterial line is in situ, avoid frequent distress from heel pricks.

- For the heel prick procedure, follow the guidance from the UK newborn blood spot sampling guidance (Public Health England, 2021).

Preparation: Any method, ensure time is appropriate for the neonate and provide comfort measures and/or procedural pain measures (sucrose, pacifier, breast milk, facilitative holding, skin to skin).

Site: Ensure correct site is ascertained. For heel prick, see Chapter 4, Figure 4.1.

Taking blood: Blood should be collected as quickly as possible to prevent clotting, avoiding prolonged squeezing which may affect the result.

 Standard precautions alert

Remember to wear gloves when taking and handling blood and observe careful handwashing before and after.

 Check local guidance

Check the national guidance for heel pricks, as well as the local guidance on blood sampling procedures.

Stop and think

Caution should be taken in how much blood is taken for repeat tests. This should be monitored, particularly in very small neonates whose blood volume can easily be depleted.

Giving blood in the neonatal unit

A blood transfusion may be required in the neonate for the prevention of anaemia secondary to prematurity or blood loss, when the haemoglobin (Hb) drops to an operational threshold level (subject to local guidelines on low acceptable values). According to Sweet et al (2023), the recommendation is that thresholds for red blood cell transfusion in infants can be set at 12 g/dL (haematocrit (HCT) 36%) for those with severe cardio-respiratory disease, 11 g/dL (HCT 30%) for those who are oxygen dependent, and 7 g/dL (HCT 25%) for stable infants beyond two weeks of age. Table 11.8 outlines a guide with practice points for giving blood transfusions.

⊞ Table 11.8 Giving blood in the neonatal unit

Blood product	Indication and threshold for transfusion
Packed cells	**For anaemia/blood loss** Transfuse if symptomatic. If reticulocytes >1%, a transfusion may not be necessary
Platelets	**For thrombocytopenia** Infant who is unwell/bleeding
Fresh frozen plasma (FFP)	**For prolonged clotting time (PTT)**
Cryoprecipitate	**For low fibrinogen**

CARDIOVASCULAR CARE

A healthy neonate who has a clear airway and is breathing effectively will be well perfused with a cardiovascular system (CVS) able to deliver all essential nutrients and oxygen to the body. However, in the sick neonate who does not have the compensatory mechanisms to cope with compromise, support for the CVS is often necessary. This section covers an overview of CVS care (Tables 11.9 to 11.11 and Figure 11.16).

Cardiovascular system monitoring

 Table 11.9 Monitoring of the cardiovascular system

CVS compromise and poor tissue perfusion is indicated by:

- tachycardia;
- capillary refill time (CRT) >3 seconds;
- metabolic acidosis – eg lactate >2 mmol/L and/or base excess < minus 8 mmol/L with normal chloride;
- oliguria <1 ml/kg/hour, especially after 24 hours of age;
- hypotension – low mean blood pressure (MBP <30 mmHg).*

*A general agreement for MBP for the first few days of life is gestation in weeks. However, in practice, a MBP less than 30 mmHg is often the acceptable lower limit used and giving fluid volume may be considered at this point (Yates and Rennie, 2014).

Monitor arterial blood pressure, heart rate, CRT, blood gases (lactate and base excess) and urine output. Also, ensure adequate oxygen saturations, other blood gas values, glucose and respiratory function/lung expansion.

Monitor MBP continually via arterial line or by regular cuff readings.

Table 11.10 Management of cardiovascular system compromise

Aim: To improve cardiac output and perfusion of vital organs to prevent shock.

- Treatment of hypotension is recommended when there is evidence of poor tissue perfusion such as oliguria, acidosis and poor capillary refill. Treatment will depend on the cause (Sweet et al, 2023).
- Labour room resuscitation care may include respiratory support, intravenous volume and/or blood, sodium bicarbonate,* glucose or adrenaline.
- Overall, therapeutic interventions include volume, inotropes and/or steroids.
- **Volume:** 10 to 20 ml/kg saline or blood products if there is clear evidence of blood loss – eg antepartum haemorrhage (APH), abruption, severe pallor, low packed cell volume.
- **Inotropes:** dobutamine, dopamine, adrenaline.
- **Corticosteroids** can be considered in conjunction with above therapies.

* Sodium bicarbonate correction (<u>to correct metabolic acidosis</u>)

Compromise due to a patent ductus arteriosus (PDA)

This leads to CVS instability, including drops in blood pressure and difficulty weaning from the ventilator/respiratory support.

When a decision is made to attempt pharmacological closure of hemodynamically significant PDA, indomethacin, ibuprofen or paracetamol can be used with a similar efficacy. Paracetamol is preferred when there is thrombocytopenia or concerns about renal function (Sweet et al, 2023).

See the web companion for more detailed explanations of cardiovascular compromise due to cardiac failure, the presence of a patent ductus arteriosus and other cardiac conditions.

 Stop and think

- Caution should be applied when administering fluid volumes to a neonate as kidney function is immature. The risk of overload should be guarded against.

- The potential risks of drugs used to increase blood pressure should be considered and close monitoring undertaken.

- For inotrope administration, care should be taken in titrating doses to avoid rapid swings in blood pressure that can affect brain perfusion.

- Caution should be applied with the administration of sodium bicarbonate and steroid use due to the potential serious side effects.

Monitoring blood pressure

Careful and regular assessment is necessary when the CVS is accessed by the arterial system for blood sampling and monitoring of the circulation.

 Table 11.11 Monitoring blood pressure in neonates

- Assist with arterial line insertion and safe securing via umbilical artery (UAC) or other peripheral artery access – see Figure 11.16.
- Set up infusion system with heparinised saline through an arterial-giving set including a transducer. Ensure the correct waveform scale is chosen for blood pressure on the monitor. Calibrate the system to zero prior to commencing monitoring (and calibrate each shift).
- Arterial alarms should be checked on set-up and at the beginning of each shift.
- If there is no arterial access, take regular cuff readings (hourly or as indicated by the neonate's condition), manually or automatically timed.

 Standard precautions alert

Standard precautions must be observed during set-up of the arterial line system to prevent introduction of infection to the neonate as well as to protect oneself from blood. The infusion fluid, transducer set and three-way tap should be changed according to local policy.

Stop and think

Safety: Close and regular observation of arterial and umbilical lines should be maintained to prevent the associated risks such as bleeding, blockage by a blood clot and the effect on perfusion. Check/observe limbs for perfusion – colour, circulation, pulse and temperature of extremity distal to the puncture site. The line may need to be removed if perfusion is compromised. See the web companion for detail on UAC care.

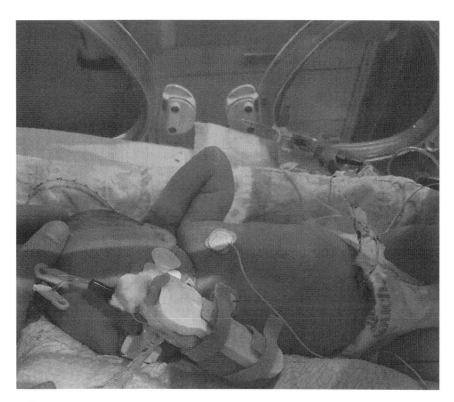

Figure 11.16 Infant with a UAC in situ

DRUG ADMINISTRATION

It is an essential part of safe nursing practice to be able to calculate and administer drugs correctly and to understand their dosage, indications and side effects. This is particularly important in neonatal care as we are dealing with a distinct group of smaller, vulnerable patients. It is beyond the scope of this book to do justice to all potential drugs administered in the neonatal unit along with varying calculation examples – therefore, the reader is referred to the web companion. What is included below are some useful formulas to familiarise oneself with for safe neonatal medication practice (Table 11.12).

 Stop and think

Neonatal drug dosages are more likely to be prescribed and given in micrograms than larger units, compared to older age groups. Certain drugs are also given in nanograms. It is very important to understand how to convert larger units to smaller units for accuracy and to avoid errors in administration.

 See the web companion for further information on drugs and drug calculations.

 Table 11.12 Understanding strengths, units and formulas

a – Converting grams to milligrams to micrograms to nanograms.
(Multiply by 1000 to convert larger unit to smaller units)
Grams (g) to milligrams (mg) – multiply by 1000.
Milligrams (mg) to micrograms (mcg) – multiply by 1000.
Micrograms (mcg) to nanograms (ng) – multiply by 1000.
Converting nanograms to micrograms to milligrams to grams
(Divide by 1000 each time to convert smaller to larger units)
b – 1 in 1000, 1 in 10,000
(Parts of an active drug in a given volume)
1 in 1000 means 1 g in 1000 ml (1000 mg in 1000 ml = 1 mg per ml)
1 in 10,000 means 1 g in 10,000 ml (ie less concentrated)
1000 mg in 10,000 ml = 1 mg in 10 ml
c – mmol – eg for sodium bicarbonate, electrolytes
Molarity refers to atomic weight.
1 mole is the molecular weight for a drug.
mmol is one thousandth of a mole
d – Units of activity
Eg for drugs from natural sources such as heparin (1000 units in 1 ml), insulin (100 units in 1 ml) or hormones

e – How many grams in a certain %?

Strength as a percentage means the number of parts per hundred

5% glucose is 5 parts glucose in 100 parts of volume (5 g in 100 ml)

10% glucose is 10 parts glucose in 100 parts (10 g in 100 ml)

Useful formulas

Giving a drug – How much do I need to draw up?

Volume needed =

$$\frac{\text{What you want}}{\text{What you've got}} \times \text{volume the drug is in}$$

You should check that both the dose prescribed and the drug being used are the same in units (eg milligrams)

Calculating doses from infusion rates

Quantity of drug put into syringe (in mcg or ng)*

Divided by the volume in the syringe

Divided by the neonate's weight**

Multiplied by the infusion rate running

This gives you the dose in <u>mcg/kg/hour</u> (being given by the current rate of infusion)

* Convert mg to mcg first (multiply mg × 1000 to get the drug in mcg) or convert to ng

**NB if the drug (eg inotropes) is given in mcg/kg/<u>minute</u> SO ALSO divide by 60 at this point <u>In other words</u>:

The initial dose (mcgs) *divided by* the weight (kg) *divided by* the volume (ml) gives you *<u>the dose per kg per hour</u> in 1 ml.* You then multiply by the final figure by the current rate of infusion

Divide this by 60 (minutes) to give you the dose *<u>per kg per minute</u>*

 Stop and think

Some drug infusions are calculated in mcg/kg/hour, while others are in mcg/kg/minute depending on the half-life of the drug being given. It is important to know this when checking the prescription and calculate accordingly.

See the web companion for more complex/specialised areas of care and specific conditions, namely, surgical care, neurological care including hypoxic ischaemic encephalopathy, intraventricular haemorrhage, neonatal abstinence syndrome and neonatal transport. The web companion also includes a glossary specific to this chapter.

🔴 Check local variations and guidance alert

The space below can be used to record any notes or local variations and practice points specific to your own unit.

REFERENCES

Arias-Oliveras, A (2016) Neonatal Blood Gas Interpretation. *Newborn and Infant Nursing Reviews*, 16(3): 119–21.

Chang, D W (2011) *Respiratory Care Calculations*. 3rd ed. Albany, NY: Delmar.

National Institute for Health and Care Excellence (NICE) (2019) Specialist Neonatal Respiratory Care for Babies Born Preterm. NICE Guideline [NG124]. [online] Available at: www.nice.org.uk/guidance/ng124 (accessed 1 November 2023).

Petty, J (2013) Understanding Neonatal Ventilation: Strategies for Decision Making in the NICU. *Neonatal Network*, 32(4): 246–61.

Public Health England (2021) Newborn Blood Spot Sampling Guidelines: Quick Reference Guide. [online] Available at: www.gov.uk/government/publications/newborn-blood-spot-screening-sampling-guidelines/quick-reference-guide (accessed 31 October 2023).

Rennie, J (2012) *Rennie & Roberton's Textbook of Neonatology E-Book*. Churchill Livingstone.

Sweet, D G, Carnielli, V P, Greisen, G et al (2023) European Consensus Guidelines on the Management of Respiratory Distress Syndrome: 2022 Update. *Neonatology*, 120(1): 3–23.

UK Resuscitation Council (2021) *Newborn Resuscitation and Support of Transition of Infants at Birth Guidelines*. [online] Available at: www.resus.org.uk/library/2021-resuscitation-guidelines/newborn-resuscitation-and-support-transition-infants-birth (accessed 5 December 2023).

Yates, R and Rennie, J M (2014) *Appendix 4: Normal Values for Neonatal Blood Pressure – Expert Consult*. [online] Available at: https://obgynkey.com/normal-values-for-neonatal-blood-pressure (accessed 5 December 2023).

12 Principles of family integrated care in the neonatal unit

Louise McLaughlin and Julia Petty

INTRODUCTION

Admission to the neonatal unit has significant psychosocial implications for parents. There are several family-focused interventions that health professionals can deliver that help reduce the stress experienced by parents in the neonatal unit (Fowler et al, 2019; Petty et al, 2019; Hirtz et al, 2023). Vital components of family integrated care (FICare) relating to emotional and psychosocial care of the family are detailed in Figures 12.1 to 12.3 and Table 12.1. Figures 12.4 and 12.5 focus on partnership and empowerment and recognising diversity for inclusive practice, respectively. The chapter continues with an inclusion of ethical decision-making and end-of-life care in Tables 12.2 and 12.3 and Figure 12.6. These are all interconnecting aspects of care that are fundamental to the optimum psycho-emotional support of the family in the neonatal unit.

Chapter learning objectives

By the end of this chapter you will:

✓ be able to identify the five principles of family integrated care and how they are applied in an inclusive way to the care of the family;

✓ have gained an overview of the requirements of caring for a neonate with palliative care needs on the neonatal unit.

Critical thinking points

• How can the implementation of family integrated care differ between the individual needs of families, considering inclusivity?

• How can the palliative care needs and wishes for a neonate and their family be met while on the neonatal unit?

See Chapter 6 and Chapter 9 on key issues relating to the family. See also the web companion for supplementary information.

FAMILY INTEGRATED CARE

Family integrated care (FICare) is a collaborative model of neonatal care which aims to address the negative impacts of the neonatal intensive care unit (NICU) environment by involving parents as equal partners, minimising separation and supporting parent–infant closeness (Waddington et al, 2021) (Figures 12.1 to 12.3).

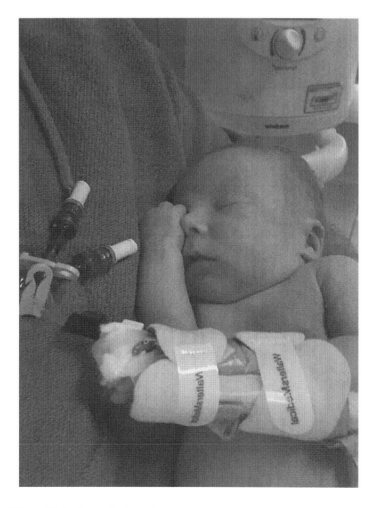

Figure 12.1 Neonate held by parent

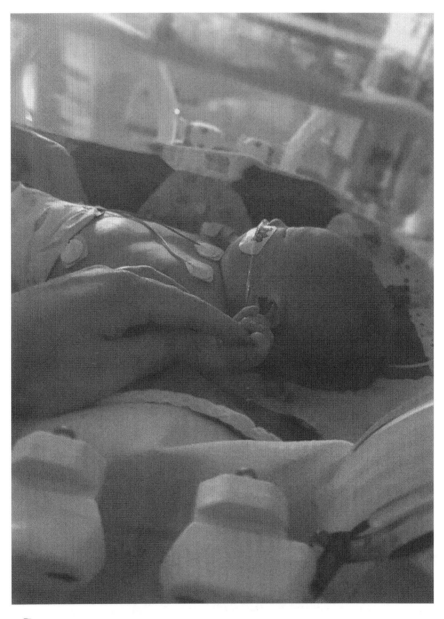

Figure 12.2 Parent with hand on their neonate

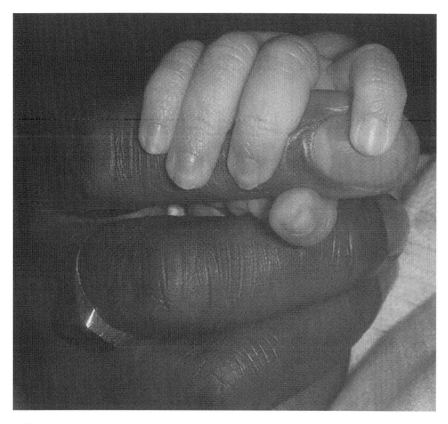

 Figure 12.3 Neonate and father holding hands

⊞ Table 12.1 Family integrated care (FICare) principles (British Association of Perinatal Medicine (BAPM), 2021; Bliss, 2023)

Charter principle	How the principle is upheld
Partnerships with families – *Families are equal partners in the care team and are included in all aspects of their babies' care, including shared decision making.*	✓ Families are encouraged to become involved in their babies' care as primary caregivers. ✓ If a high-risk pregnancy is anticipated to result in a neonatal admission, the families should be supported and encouraged to be comfortable providing care for their babies from the point of diagnosis. ✓ Families are encouraged to participate in ward rounds, daily care planning and decision making. ✓ Families have opportunities to give feedback about their babies' care while on the unit and after discharge. ✓ Families' experiences and feedback are actively sought to inform and improve the quality of services.

→

Table 12.1 (cont.)

Charter principle	How the principle is upheld
Empowerment – *Families are equipped to engage fully in their babies' needs through education and training.*	✓ Families are orientated to the neonatal unit environment on admission or if an admission was anticipated during pregnancy, then at the point of diagnosis. ✓ Families have a clear understanding of their role as caregivers as well as the principles of family integrated care. ✓ Families are aware of what support services are available during their stay, including those available through charities. ✓ Families receive ongoing teaching and support, which is tailor made to the baby and family. ✓ Family classes and activities offered in a flexible and convenient way for families, which may include evenings and weekends and peer-to-peer learning
Well-being – *Family mental health and welfare are priorities as well as staff well-being.*	✓ Specialist psychological and mental health support should be available during admission and after discharge for families as well as staff. ✓ Family-based activities should be available for families both on the unit and in the community. This includes activities such as peer-to-peer support. ✓ The neonatal unit should consider the role of a family liaison officer. ✓ There should be inclusive and equitable access for all families, including translation of written literature and the use of translators on the unit. ✓ Liaise with community groups and charities who can provide well-being support for families.
Culture – *Neonatal units adopt a culture that promotes integration of families into the delivery of care.*	✓ All neonatal team members should receive training on the philosophy and benefits of FICare. ✓ All staff should be clear of the expectations of their practice to support families. ✓ Additional training should be provided to staff in the provision of developmentally supportive care, neurodevelopmental care and trauma-informed care. ✓ Multi-disciplinary FICare 'champions' should be identified to support the changes in practice.

Charter principle	How the principle is upheld
Environment – *Neonatal units should promote a physical and social environment that allows parents to spend as much time as they would like with their babies.*	✓ The neonatal unit environment should be welcoming for all families. Provisions should include a dedicated family room, kitchen facilities for heating and storing food and personal storage space. There should also be a dedicated room for mothers to breastfeed if privacy is required. ✓ The unit should encourage 24-hour open access for families to be with their babies. ✓ The cot-side environment should meet the families' needs, with access to reclining chairs, breast pumps and screens for privacy. ✓ Families should have clear signposting to financial support. ✓ Play therapists should be available to support siblings while on the unit. ✓ Rooming-in facilities should be available for families to aid transition to home discharge. ✓ Babies receiving end-of-life care should do so in a dedicated room.
Inclusion of the Bliss Baby Charter Principles	✓ The Bliss Baby Charter is recognised as a key tool in BAPM's framework for FICare practice. ✓ The seven Baby Charter Principles – social and developmental needs; decision making; staff and services; benchmarking; unit facilities; feeding; and discharge – align firmly with FICare principles of family partnership, empowerment, culture, environment and well-being.

Refer to the BAPM (2021) document for full guidance and the Bliss Baby Charter (2023)

(Adapted from British Association of Perinatal Medicine, 2021; Bliss, 2023)

 Stop and think

All parents should be encouraged and supported to be involved in planning and providing care, ensuring that communication with clinical staff occurs throughout the care pathway. An inclusive approach to the care of parents is essential – to include all cultures, ethnicities, social situations, sexual orientation, gender identity, age, disability and neurodiversity with care and communication tailored accordingly.

Negotiate individualised care plan with the parents

Communicate to parents how to be involved in their neonate's care and agree strategies

PARTNERSHIP FOR EMPOWERMENT

Involve parents in any decision making about their neonate

Facilitate and support parental involvement in care as much as possible, to empower their parenting role

 Figure 12.4 Partnership and negotiation

 Stop and think

To ensure the principles of family integrated care can be delivered, information sharing must not be a one-way communication. Understanding the parents' personal values and preferences is important to reach shared understanding and decision making (Brødsgaard et al, 2019)

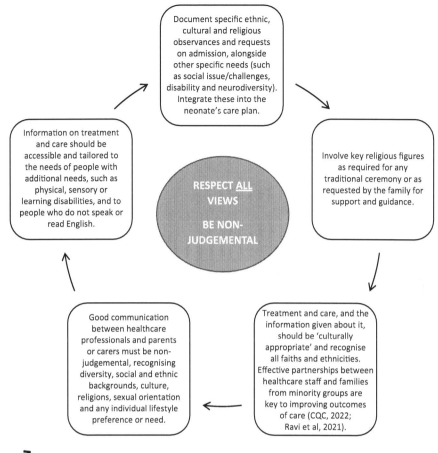

Figure 12.5 Guide to recognising diversity and culturally appropriate care

 Stop and think

Recognising diversity and avoiding discrimination is an essential component of lawful care of any patient (Equality Act 2010). Observation of the cultural elements of family and personal life is an essential consideration (Holland, 2018) and should be considered throughout a family's stay in the neonatal unit.

ETHICAL DECISION MAKING IN THE NEONATAL UNIT

Care of the family as an overarching term includes the principles of sound, family-focused ethical decision making. This is particularly important in the field of palliative care and when outcomes of sick neonates are not expected to be favourable. This is a vital area of consideration given the potential complexities of neonatal care, advances in technology and the increasing number of extremely preterm neonates surviving neonatal care. Around 2000 babies each year are admitted to the neonatal unit in England and Wales with palliative care needs (Harden et al, 2023). Therefore, certain care practices can involve complex and often-sensitive dilemmas, raising ethical debates that require clarity for staff and parents to make sense of such issues. Examples presented here are the issues of obtaining consent and upholding confidentiality in the neonatal unit (Table 12.2), followed by the delicate subject of withdrawing or withholding life-sustaining treatment in the sick and vulnerable neonate (Figure 12.6). End-of-life care then follows to end this chapter (Table 12.3).

 Table 12.2 Ethical–legal issues relating to parents in the neonatal unit: practice points

---

Maintaining confidentiality

- Confidentiality is a legal obligation for all healthcare staff caring for neonates and their families.

- Person-identifiable information regarding the neonate and family must be protected against disclosure (includes talking about patients in public places where they can be overheard, leaving any information lying around unattended and leaving computer terminals logged in allowing open access to files).

- Access to confidential information must be on a need-to-know basis and limited to the purpose for which it is required.

- Any decision to disclose information about the neonate and family must be justified, in their best interest and should be documented clearly.

(Taken from NHS England, 2019; refer to this document for full guidance.)

Obtaining consent

- Consent may be obtained for clinical interventions, post-mortem examination or research participation. Where possible, all procedures should be explained.

- Consent may be written, verbal or implied. For the more serious, invasive procedures however, consent is written, and is essential for verbal consent to be combined with clear documentation, supported by a parental signature that is witnessed.

- Consent should be obtained by whoever is undertaking the procedure and/or someone who is trained appropriately.

- Nurses should witness and be involved in any meeting where consent is obtained.

- Documentation is a vital component of consent, particularly parental understanding and agreement of a procedure or procedures.

- In neonatal care, consent is obtained from someone with parental responsibility (parents if married, mother but not father if unmarried unless there is a parental responsibility agreement or the father is named on the birth certificate).

- Consent is valid only if information is understood by the parents – this includes why an intervention is necessary, as well as the risks and implications.

- It is good practice in neonatal care to communicate clearly from as early as possible from neonatal admission, including provision of written information where possible.

- In addition, cultural and religious factors must be considered when discussing options for interventions which may impact on parental decisions to give consent.

 Check local guidance

Observe any local guidance and advice along with national guidelines on any ethical–legal matters in the neonatal unit.

 Stop and think

It is a legal and ethical requirement to gain valid consent before *any* investigation for any patient at any age. However, exceptions apply; it is not usually necessary to document consent to routine interventions that are part of the daily care of the neonate and in emergency situations it may not be possible to obtain parental consent. In this case, treatment can be given if it is deemed *in the best interest* of the neonate.

The decision to withdraw/withhold treatment

The decision is taken when it is deemed that continuing treatment is *not in the best interests of the neonate* and to continue such would cause prolonged suffering and distress. (For full ethical guidance, see Royal College of Paediatrics and Child Health (RCPCH, 2015) and the Nuffield Council on Bioethics (2006).)

Once a decision has been made (see full guidance by Mancini et al, 2014)

- Ensure both parents, if applicable, are present for any discussions in a private room along with members of their support network such as family members, friends, religious figures.
- A time and location (eg, hospital, hospice, or home) for withdrawal of care is agreed with consideration of the likelihood of death during transfer to hospice/home and the uncertainty of length of time to death.
- Parents should be supported while the withdrawal of treatment occurs. Their wishes should be outlined in the baby's Advance Care Plan but may include such things as holding their baby, playing music, or acknowledging religious or cultural traditions.

Physical considerations

Pain relief	Physiological monitoring	Symptom control	Fluids and nutrition	Ventilation and oxygen
Assess pain. Prescribe analgesia, preferably IV route or subcutaneous/ buccal/enteral as tolerated. Employ non-pharmacological conform measures.	Discontinue invasive interventions and blood tests. Monitor for signs of discomfort.	Assess and treat distressing symptoms appropriately. Anticipatory symptoms should be considered in a symptom management plan.	Continue to maintain comfort unless feeding causes pain and distress, then the decision is reviewed.	Removal of ETT and cessation of ventilation support is done when fully agreed with the family. Oxygen may be offered as symptom management.

Psychosocial considerations

Religious and spiritual	Psychological support
Assess and integrate religious/spiritual needs, including key religious figures and rituals as requested. This should be outlined in the Advance Care Plan.	Liaise with the multi-disciplinary team – eg, psychologists, counsellors. Needs will vary. Offer appropriate choices.

The GOAL of care is COMFORT

 Figure 12.6 Withholding or withdrawing treatment in the neonatal unit: overview of selected key points

 Stop and think

The decision process to withdraw/withhold treatment can take considerable time and deliberation within the whole team, *including the parents*. The nurse and doctor caring for the neonate should be present at any discussions as well as the palliative care team and, if appropriate, the community or outreach teams. Any conflicts in decision making need resolution to move forward.

⊞ Table 12.3 Perinatal pathway for babies with palliative care needs

Stage 1 – Eligibility for the perinatal pathway

- Sharing significant news – families should be told of their babies' prognosis in a timely manner using sensitive but effective communication. This news may be shared antenatally, during birth or after the baby has been born.

- Plan for location of care – families should be offered a choice of where they would like their child to be cared for, including where the mother may give birth, in order for the family to have an opportunity to spend time together. The choice of location needs to be realistic and appropriate for mother and baby's needs.

Stage 2 – Ongoing care

- Multi-agency assessment of families' needs – this should be an ongoing assessment, examining all factors that impact the baby's and family's quality of life, guiding the delivery of care.

- Co-ordinated multi-agency care plans – these should include parallel planning and may cover the antenatal period, delivery and postnatal care, looking at health, social, religious and spiritual care. An advance care plan and symptom management plan are good examples of this when clearly linked together. Care plans can be reviewed at any time. Resuscitation plans should be considered.

Stage 3 – End-of-life and bereavement care

- End-of-life care plan – parents should be supported when discussing their chosen place of death for their baby as well as in making memories with their baby, including support for siblings, grandparents, aunts and uncles. Families should have access to a 24-hour palliative care team, medication and equipment. Consideration of the need for a post-mortem or organ donation should be discussed. The family should be offered time with their baby post death, with the option to be involved in the care of the body such as washing and dressing; this may involve moving the baby to a different location such as a cold bedroom in a children's hospice.

- Bereavement care – bereavement support should be offered on assessed needs with consideration of local and national sources of support. The needs of siblings should also be considered. All families should be offered a follow-up appointment with their consultant or care team to reflect and ask questions. Any support around future pregnancies should be considered.

(Together for Short Lives (TFSL), 2017; National Institute for Health and Care Excellence (NICE), 2019)

 Stop and think

Palliative care is a total approach to care from the point of diagnosis or recognition of a life-limiting or life-threatening condition. It embraces, physical, social, emotional and spiritual elements (TFSL, 2017).

See the web companion for a glossary specific to this chapter.

 Check local variations and guidance alert

The space below can be used to record any notes or local variations and practice points specific to your own unit.

REFERENCES

Bliss (2023) What Is the Baby Charter? [online] Available at: www.bliss.org.uk/health-professionals/bliss-baby-charter/what-is-the-baby-charter (accessed 5 December 2023).

British Association of Perinatal Medicine (BAPM) (2021) *Family Integrated Care: A Framework for Practice.* [online] Available at: www.bapm.org/resources/ficare-framework-for-practice (accessed 5 December 2023).

Brødsgaard, A, Pedersen, J T, Larsen, P and Weis, J (2019) Parents' and Nurses' Experiences of Partnership in Neonatal Intensive Care Units: A Qualitative Review and Meta-Synthesis. *Journal of Clinical Nursing*, 28(17–18): 3117–39.

Care Quality Commission (CQC) (2022) Culturally Appropriate Care. [online] Available at: www.cqc.org.uk/guidance-providers/adult-social-care/culturally-appropriate-care (accessed 28 January 2024).

Equality Act 2010. [online] Available at: www.legislation.gov.uk/ukpga/2010/15/contents (accessed 5 December 2023).

Fowler, C, Green, J, Whiting, L, Petty, J, Rossiter, C and Elliott, D (2019) The Forgotten Mothers of Extremely Preterm Babies: Need for Increased Psychosocial Support. *Journal of Clinical Nursing*, 8(11–12): 2124–34.

Harden, F, Lanoue, J, Modi, N, Uthaya S N and Battersby, C (2023) Data-Driven Approach to Understanding Neonatal Palliative Care Needs in England and Wales: A Population-Based Study 2015–2020. *Archives of Disease in Childhood. Fetal and Neonatal Edition*, 108(5): 540–4.

Hirtz, K, Lau, M, Hall, A and Fucile, S (2023) Interventions Aimed at Reducing the Stress of Mothers Whose Infant Is Born Premature: A Scoping Review. *Journal of Neonatal Nursing*, 29(4): 602–11.

Holland, K (2018) *Cultural Awareness in Nursing and Health Care: An Introductory Text*. 3rd ed. London: Routledge.

Mancini, A, Uthaya, S, Beardsley, C, Wood, D and Modi, N (2014) *Practical Guidance for the Management of Palliative Care on Neonatal Units*. 1st ed. [online] Available at: www.chelwest.nhs.uk/services/childrens-services/neonatal-services/links/Practical-guidance-for-the-management-of-palliative-care-on-neonatal-units-Feb-2014.pdf (accessed 5 December 2023).

National Institute for Health and Care Excellence (NICE) (2019) *End of Life Care for Infants, Children and Young People with Life-Limiting Conditions: Planning and Management Recommendations*. London: NICE.

NHS England (2019) *Confidentiality Policy*. London: NHS England.

Nuffield Council on Bioethics (2006) *Critical Care Decisions in Fetal and Neonatal Medicine: Ethical Issues*. [online] Available at: http://nuffieldbioethics.org/wp-content/uploads/2014/07/CCD-web-version-22-June-07-updated.pdf (accessed 5 December 2023).

Petty, J, Jarvis, J and Thomas, R (2019) Understanding Parents' Emotional Experiences for Neonatal Education: A Narrative, Interpretive Approach. *Journal of Clinical Nursing*, 28(9–10): 1911–24.

Ravi, D, Iacob, A and Profit, J (2021) Unequal Care: Racial/ethnic Disparities in Neonatal Intensive Care Delivery. *Seminars in Perinatology*, 45(4). 10.1016/j.semperi.2021.151411.

Royal College of Paediatrics and Child Health (2015) Making Decisions to Limit Treatment in Life-Limiting and Life-Threatening Conditions in Children: A Framework for Practice. *Archive of Diseases in Childhood*, 100(suppl 2): 1–26.

Together for Short Lives (TFSL) (2017) *A Perinatal Pathway for Babies with Palliative Care Needs*. 2nd ed. [online] Available at: www.togetherforshortlives.org.uk/app/uploads/2018/01/ProRes-Perinatal-Pathway-for-Babies-With-Palliative-Care-Needs.pdf (accessed 5 December 2023).

Waddington, C, van Veenendaal, N R, O'Brien, K and Patel, N for the International Steering Committee for Family Integrated Care (2021) Family Integrated Care: Supporting Parents as Primary Caregivers in the Neonatal Intensive Care Unit. *Pediatric Investigation*, 15(2): 148–54.

Part 3

Caring for the vulnerable neonate at and after discharge

Section editors: Sheila Roberts and Lisa Whiting

13 Planning for discharge and caring for the infant at home

Lisa Whiting

INTRODUCTION

Thorough discharge planning, which starts when the infant is admitted to the neonatal unit, is fundamental to the smooth transition home. Discharge planning needs to adopt a two-way communication strategy that enables a range of health professionals to provide parents with support that embraces educational, medical and emotional aspects of care. High-quality discharge planning means that parents are far more likely to feel able to look after their infant in the home environment, confident in the knowledge that they know who to contact should the need arise. This chapter discusses the specific areas that need to be considered, both prior to discharge and when the infant is at home (Tables 13.1 to 13.5).

Chapter learning objectives

By the end of this chapter you will:

✓ understand why early and thorough discharge planning is crucial to the smooth transition from the neonatal unit to the home environment, for both parent and infant;

✓ be able to identify support strategies for parents when caring for their infant in the home environment.

Critical thinking points

- How would you facilitate appropriate discharge planning and the smooth transition home for the infant and their family?

- What are the key facilitators that enable parents to confidently care for their infant at home, post discharge from the neonatal unit?

See also Chapter 15 on community care relating to the family.

 See also the web companion for supplementary information relating to this chapter.

PLANNING FOR DISCHARGE HOME

Taking an infant home, who has been cared for in a neonatal unit, can be an exciting but also a very daunting prospect. Discharge planning involves working with the family to ensure that the transition home is smooth and successful; it should start at the point of admission (Smith et al, 2022), with several aspects being central to its preparation (Table 13.1).

 Table 13.1 Key considerations for discharge planning from the neonatal unit to home

---

Discharge planning should:

- start from the infant's point of admission to the neonatal unit;

- be a continuous process;

- involve both informal and formal education;

- acknowledge the specific circumstances of each parent (including individual, family and social situations);

- focus on the specific needs of the individual infant;

- consider the infant's clinical condition as well as how the parent(s) adapt to the circumstances;

- embrace physical and emotional aspects;

- consider how the smooth transition home can be facilitated;

- be extended to the wider family.

(Osorio Galeano and Salazar Maya, 2023)

 Stop and think

It is easy to underestimate the complexity of discharge planning and the range of elements involved. It is time-consuming, requiring continuity and excellent communication strategies.

One of the initial priorities is to build parental confidence so that they not only feel able to competently carry out daily care when at home but know who to contact should a health problem arise. It is important to get to know the parent(s) throughout the infant's stay in the neonatal unit, documenting key points in the notes so that these can be referred to as discharge nears and discussions become more focused (for example, a parent may mention that they live in a high-rise flat and that the lift is frequently 'out of order' – knowing this will enable bespoke information to be provided). As discharge approaches (a minimum of 48 hours beforehand, but longer if possible), it is important to have a discussion with the parent(s) about their concerns and anxieties. Although parents may have older children, they may be very anxious about taking their vulnerable infant home; it is useful to make a list of areas that parents would like further advice about and these can then be added to the neonatal unit's generic checklist. It is also crucial to involve the rest of the family, especially siblings and grandparents (the latter of whom may be involved in day-to-day care activities when parents return to work). Therefore, talk to parents about who is important in their lives and who may benefit from being included in the discharge planning.

The date of discharge will be influenced by a number of factors but primarily the infant's physical readiness; in addition, the timing needs to be as convenient as possible for the parent(s); for example, it may be that if an infant is discharged home towards the end of a working week, there are other family members who can provide support during the initial few days at home, especially if they span a weekend (this may be even more imperative if a parent has had a multiple birth such as twins). Having a date goal to aim for also facilitates the organisation of the discharge planning arrangements.

TRANSITION FROM HOSPITAL TO HOME

Smith et al (2022) offer guidelines to facilitate discharge planning and the transition home, highlighting four key areas.

o *Basic information*: this refers to the knowledge that every family will require, irrespective of their individual and specific needs; it includes discharge education, planning tools, the team and the process.

o *Anticipatory guidance*: this focuses on parents developing a good insight into what life will be like when they are at home with their infant.

o *Transfer and co-ordination of care*: this centres on the transition of care from the acute neonatal unit to the community.

o *Other important considerations*: this encompasses factors that may be specific to individual families and where there may be particular needs; examples include families where there is limited command of the English language, those who have disabilities, those from an LGBTQIA+ background and those in the military; but there are, of course, other circumstances too, such as: disabled (physical and learning disabilities) and neurodiverse parents, young parents/ teenagers and those from socially deprived areas who may have socio-financial challenges.

Further details of the above areas are provided in Table 13.2.

⊞ Table 13.2 Summary of the four key areas of discharge planning and transition home

Aspect	Interpretation
Basic information	Discharge education that includes: • feeding; • bathing; • dressing – day and night; • how to change a nappy and the frequency to be expected; • home medication information; • provision of a safe sleeping position and environment; • how to recognise illness, including a pyrexia; • protecting the infant from infections; • use of any technology that may be used at home; • basic life support education; • information about immunisations; • preparing the home environment (for example, safety measures); • the journey home (for example, an appropriate car seat); • thinking of the help that parents may need once home. Discharge planning tools that include: • a comprehensive discharge summary; • supplementary educational materials, such as resources produced by the neonatal unit or charities (for example, Bliss). Discharge planning team that may involve: • nurses, doctors, psychologists, social workers, advance nurse practitioners; • those who will be involved in the infant's care at home; • siblings. Discharge planning process that: • starts on the infant's admission to the neonatal unit and continues throughout their stay; • provides clear and consistent messages.

Aspect	Interpretation
Anticipatory guidance	Factors to be considered are: • the anticipated number of medical/clinical appointments (these could include, for example, audiology, ophthalmology, cerebral scans, physiotherapy, neonatal/paediatric/community consultant, developmental checks, immunisations); • developmental milestones and growth; • parental feelings about going home with their infant – this includes excitement, but also anxiety about caring for their infant by themselves without the infrastructure of the neonatal unit; • how to deal with a crying infant; • the type of atypical behaviour that might be encountered; • parental mental health; • potential financial implications; • what to do in an emergency; • assessment of family risk factors.
Transfer and co-ordination of care	Factors to be considered are: • involvement of primary carers; • neonatal unit contact with the family post discharge home; • community resources – who and what is available to support the transition home? • parental emotional and mental health well-being.
Other important considerations	Factors to be addressed are: • whether there is a need for an interpreter and/or computer-related services; • the potential need for additional social support; • parental literacy levels; • accessibility to services, especially if parents have disabilities; • use of terminology that is inclusive and non-discriminatory; • family beliefs.

(Adapted from Smith et al, 2022)

 Stop and think

The four areas detailed in Table 13.2 provide an overview of the key elements of discharge planning; however, the overriding factor is the individual family and ensuring that their specific needs are met.

Prior to the family leaving the neonatal unit, it is important to ascertain that all key information has been provided and that relevant procedures/policies have been appropriately followed; to facilitate that, most neonatal units have a checklist that includes similar areas to those highlighted by Smith et al (2022).

ROOMING IN

One strategy that is advocated prior to discharge is the rooming in of parents in the neonatal unit. UNICEF United Kingdom (2022, p 13) advocates that that all parents have *'the opportunity to room in with their baby for as long as needed and to take full responsibility for their baby's care'*. This enables parents to gain confidence within a safe and secure environment. Mothers have reported that rooming in aids breastfeeding, enhances bonding as well as confidence, promotes 'ownership' of the baby and helps to foster a feeling of being a family (Bennett and Sheridan, 2005).

While the benefits of rooming in have been well documented, it is important to recognise some of the challenges associated with it – most notably, it may disrupt parental sleep patterns, meaning that at the point of discharge, parents may already feel very tired; Bennett and Sheridan (2005) also reported mothers having feelings of isolation. In addition, not all neonatal units have the facilities to support rooming in so it may not always be feasible. Finally, emphasis is frequently placed on the need for the mother to room in, but it is important to consider other family members, in particular the father or same-sex partner.

BEING AT HOME

Caring for an infant after discharge from a neonatal unit can be challenging and can mean that parents need professional support (Boykova, 2016). Research by Petty et al (2018) gained insight into the post-discharge experiences of parents in relation to their preparation for caring for their extremely premature infant at home. The study revealed five areas that parents felt were important to them (Table 13.3).

⊞ Table 13.3 Summary of findings

Research finding	Interpretation
Parental support and preparation for the transition home	Parents valued the preparation that they received for discharge home and were generally very positive about the experience. However, when discharge planning was carried out at a late stage, or was rushed, they felt unprepared – thus emphasising the need for an organised approach.

Research finding	Interpretation
Ongoing health needs of the infant	Parents reported that their infants had ongoing health needs, for example, gastro-oesophageal reflux and respiratory problems; as a result, readmission to hospital was an issue. Ongoing health needs presented other challenges, including financial difficulties, as well as impacting on their own emotional well-being.
Emotional and mental health of parents	Parents had a range of feelings about going home with their infant – these included excitement but also anxiety about caring for their infant by themselves without the infrastructure of the neonatal unit.
Uncertain outcomes	Parents were worried about what the future held in terms of their infant's health and well-being – this was particularly the case if the infant had had an incident such as a cerebral haemorrhage.
Educational needs of health professionals	Parents felt that community-based health professionals could lack knowledge and suggested a need for more focused education in terms of the specific needs of premature infants – they thought that this would facilitate a better level of support and advice for parents.

(Petty et al, 2018)

 Stop and think

Parents may face a range of challenges post discharge home; these are multi-faceted and include implications for the parent, infant and wider family.

As parents may continue to be anxious about the health and well-being of their infant when home, different members of the multi-disciplinary team may be able to support them; however, parents need to understand their various roles and know who to contact. Table 13.4 provides an overview of some of the key personnel who may be able to support the family in the ongoing care and management of their infant.

⊞ Table 13.4 Summary of those who may be able to support the family in the care of their infant at home

Personnel/organisation	Why?
General practitioner (GP)	Parents need to be reminded to register their infant with their GP as they will be the key point of contact in terms of healthcare and can also refer to other services as required.
Health visitor (HV)	The HV may already have been in contact with the family while the infant was being cared for in the neonatal unit. The HV will be able to monitor the infant's growth and development as well as offer advice about immunisations, feeding, parenting skills and home safety (including strategies to reduce the risk of sudden infant death syndrome).
Community neonatal team/ community outreach team	Some neonatal units have a team of nurses who support the transition home and who also liaise with other members of the multi-disciplinary team (such as dieticians). If the infant needs more substantive support at home, such as oxygen therapy, a community neonatal/ community outreach team is likely to be involved.
Community children's nurse (CCN)	Not all geographical areas will have a CCN team and not all parents will require access to one. However, some infants may have long-term health problems that require ongoing nursing care in the home environment (for example, respiratory problems).
Practice nurse	Parents may visit their practice nurse for their infant's immunisations.
Charities, such as Bliss (www. bliss.org.uk/about-us/what-we-do/support-families)	Charities provide a vast array of resources as well as face-to-face and email support that parents can access.

 Stop and think

The implications for families of not having appropriate advice and support must be considered as it could potentially exacerbate parental anxiety and increase the likelihood of the infant being readmitted to hospital.

In addition to professional support, parents rely heavily on social networks – this can include family members as well as friends and neighbours. This social support is extremely important, but it should be recognised that it can have both negative and positive consequences; for example, parents may receive erroneous advice that is not underpinned by sound evidence. This reinforces the need for the key people in the lives of the family to be involved in discharge planning while the infant is still in the neonatal unit. Once home, there are many causes of concern for parents, but perhaps the ones that can be most anxiety provoking are those associated with feeding, overall development, respiration and sleeping.

DEVELOPMENT

Infants who are born prematurely are at greater risk of developmental problems; examples include cerebral palsy, educational needs, motor function difficulties, speech and language development as well as learning disabilities (National Institute for Health and Care Excellence (NICE), 2017). It is therefore natural that parents may be concerned about their infant, especially as healthcare professionals may not be able to confirm whether there may be challenges ahead and/or what the severity may be. As a result, it is essential that the infant's growth and development is appropriately reviewed via an in-person consultation; during the first two years of life, NICE (2017) suggests that this is normally at the following infant-corrected ages:

o   between 3 and 5 months;

o   by 12 months;

o   at 2 years.

The assessments provide an opportunity for an in-depth discussion with the parent(s) as well as a thorough and comprehensive assessment of the infant's growth and development; a later developmental review may be undertaken at four years.

One area of development that is important to consider once the infant has been discharged home is language. Infants who are born prematurely are at a high risk of speech and communication problems; these can have a lifelong impact, both educationally and in terms of developing friendships. Despite this, little direct attention has been given to developing early language and communication skills. In a narrative-based qualitative study (Petty et al, 2023), parents reported that they had accessed information from websites, but they had little knowledge of the core components of communication beyond bonding, skin-to-skin care and direct talking and singing with their infants. One of the main barriers to parental communication with their infants was mask wearing, incubator care and conflicting advice (both in the neonatal unit and later, when at home). Therefore, there is a need for health professionals to provide ongoing, culturally appropriate post-discharge advice that supports parents to use good communication strategies that recognise their infants' cues.

Parents need to know who to get in touch with should they have concerns about any aspect of their infant's development (please refer to Table 13.4); therefore, providing a list of the names and contact details of key members of the multi-disciplinary team is very helpful.

FEEDING

One of the areas of care that can be challenging for parents to deal with in the home environment is infant feeding. Suddenly, the parent can feel isolated with no immediate access to advice or support, especially at night. Dib et al (2022) commented on the fact that challenges are common and that breastfeeding is limited in this group of infants; in their systematic review, Dib et al (2022) found that support from professionals had a significant impact on mothers' ability to exclusively breastfeed; it was suggested that an education programme (delivered while the family are in the neonatal unit) and followed up by weekly telephone contact after discharge significantly improved breastfeeding rates. Infant feeding difficulties are also extended to parents who are not able to, or who choose not to, breastfeed, and this highlights the need for regular ongoing support once the infant is at home so that parents can have any questions addressed in a timely manner. Unfortunately, this is something that can be lacking and that, as health professionals, we need to address. Petty et al (2022) found that the knowledge, skills and confidence among English health visiting students, in terms of advising and caring for parents with premature infants at home, varied and depended on individual placements and experiences. The study suggested that further education about the specific needs of premature infants and their parents was required and that more resources for community-based health professionals could optimise the support provided to parents.

Some infants may be discharged home with enteral feeding (such as a nasogastric tube), thus meaning that their length of hospital stay can potentially be reduced. Interestingly, parents may receive more support if their infant is discharged home in this situation because of the problems that can be associated with this type of nutritional support (such as tube displacement). Parents may find that they have ongoing contact with the neonatal unit and/or a community neonatal or community children's nursing team; this enables families to have a direct point of contact.

RESPIRATION

Many preterm infants may have experienced respiratory difficulties and some of these may not be fully resolved at the point of discharge. Infants requiring oxygen therapy can be safely cared for at home, providing that the family have been appropriately educated, have developed the requisite knowledge and skills and that they feel comfortable to care for their infant at home. This includes being trained in infant resuscitation prior to discharge. Bliss (nd) provide excellent resources for parents (for example *Going Home on Oxygen* and *If Your Baby is Unwell When You Go Home*) that they can be directed to. Clinical guidelines provided by the Scottish Perinatal Network Neonatal and NHS Scotland (2022) suggest that infants need to meet a set of criteria to be discharged home on oxygen (Table 13.5).

 Table 13.5 Criteria for the infant to be discharged home on oxygen

Infants should:

- be 36 weeks corrected gestational age or more;
- be physiologically stable;
- have had appropriate growth;
- have oxygen dependency of no greater than 0.5 litres per minute, via nasal cannula;
- be able to maintain an average oxygen saturation level of 93% or more;
- have had stable oxygen needs for a week;
- have had any systemic steroids stopped at least one week before;
- have had no recent changes to medication that could impact on respiration;
- be able to feed orally for a minimum of 48 hours prior to discharge (unless nasogastric feeding forms part of discharge planning);
- not have had apnoeic episodes and have had any caffeine citrate therapy discontinued for a minimum of a week;
- live in a house or flat that has been assessed and approved for suitability to have oxygen cylinders (eg appropriate access, no open fires or other hazards).

(Scottish Perinatal Network Neonatal and NHS Scotland, 2022)

 Stop and think

While the above criteria are very beneficial in terms of deciding whether an infant can be discharged home with oxygen, the ongoing needs of the parents are substantive, especially in terms of their potential anxiety levels. Think about the type of support that parents will need (and where this can be accessed from) to enable them to successfully care for their infant.

SLEEPING

While in the neonatal unit, infants may well have been exposed to an array of technology and may have become used to a range of sounds and light sources; it is not unusual for this to have an ongoing impact when they are home. It is also recognised that infants who have been born prematurely may not sleep as deeply as those born at term and that they can have more active sleep – this predisposes them to sleep difficulties. Lyu et al (2022) reported that both preterm and post-term birth infants experienced more sleeping problems, as well as a shorter sleep duration, than term infants. The type of sleep difficulties can also include those associated with breathing such as apnoea and the fact that the preterm infant has a higher risk of being a victim of sudden infant death syndrome. These factors are likely to mean that parents have heightened anxiety. In addition, it is known that the parents of preterm infants are more likely to suffer from sleep disturbances themselves because of the stress that they have experienced; this then has the potential to negatively impact on their own health and well-being (Marthinsen et al, 2018). The consequences of poor sleeping behaviours, for both the infant and parent(s), may mean that being at home is extremely challenging, especially considering the other stressors (such as infant feeding) that parents may be exposed to. As a result, parents may need to take advantage of well-being services and/or counselling – it is essential to reassure them that what they are experiencing is 'normal' so that they do not feel that they are failing in the care of their infant.

 See the web companion for a glossary specific to this chapter.

 Standard precautions alert

Teaching parents about the importance of infection prevention and signs to look out for in their infant at home is part of discharge preparation.

 Check local guidance

Check local guidance for any relevant discharge and follow-up policy.

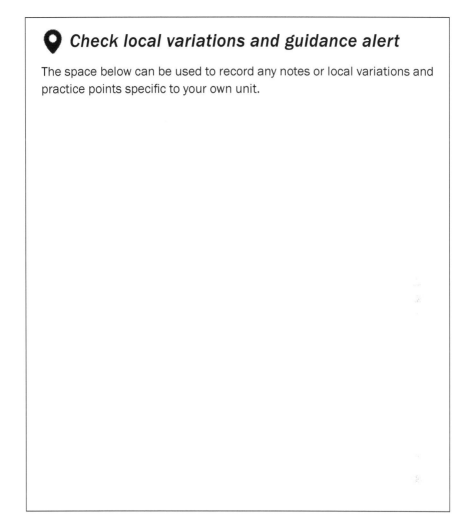

Check local variations and guidance alert

The space below can be used to record any notes or local variations and practice points specific to your own unit.

REFERENCES

Bennett, R and Sheridan, C (2005) Mothers' Perceptions of 'Rooming-In' on a Neonatal Intensive Care Unit. *Infant*, 1(5): 171–4.

Bliss (nd) Going Home on Oxygen. [online] Available at: www.bliss.org.uk/parents/going-home-from-the-neonatal-unit/going-home-on-oxygen (accessed 16 October 2023).

Bliss (nd) Resuscitation Training. [online] Available at: www.bliss.org.uk/parents/going-home-from-the-neonatal-unit/preparing-to-go-home-from-the-neonatal-unit/resuscitation-training (accessed 28 January 2024).

Boykova, M (2016) Life After Discharge: What Parents of Preterm Infants Say About Their Transition to Home. *Newborn and Infant Nursing Reviews*, 16(2): 58–65.

Dib, S, Kittisakmontri, K, Wells, J C and Fewtrell, M (2022) Interventions to Improve Breastfeeding Outcomes in Late Preterm and Early Term Infants. *Breastfeed Medicine*, 17(10): 781–92.

Lyu, J, Groeger, J A, Barnett, A L, Li, H, Wang, L, Zhang, J, Du, W and Hua, J (2022) Associations between Gestational Age and Childhood Sleep: A National Retrospective Cohort Study. *BMC Medicine*, 20: 253.

Marthinsen, G N, Helseth, S and Fegran, L (2018) Sleep and its Relationship to Health in Parents of Preterm Infants: A Scoping Review. *BMC Pediatrics*, 18(1): 352.

National Institute for Health and Care Excellence (NICE) (2017) Developmental Follow-up of Children and Young People Born Preterm. [online] Available at: www.nice.org.uk/guidance/ng72/resources/developmental-followup-of-children-and-young-people-born-preterm-pdf-1837630868677 (accessed 22 October 2023).

Osorio Galeano, S P and Salazar Maya, Á M (2023) Preparing Parents for Discharge from the Neonatal Unit, the Transition, and Care of Their Preterm Children at Home. *Investigación y Educación en Enfermería*, 41(1): e04.

Petty, J, Harding, C and Whiting, L (2023) Exploring the Parent Perspective on the Enablers and Barriers to Communication with Their Preterm Infants: A Narrative Study. *Journal of Child Health.* In press.

Petty, J, Whiting, L, Green, J, Fowler, C, Rossiter, C and Elliott, D (2018) Parents' Views on Preparation to Care for Extremely Premature Infants at Home. *Nursing Children and Young People*, 30(4): 22–7.

Petty, J, Whiting, L, Green, J and Fowler, C (2022) Exploring the Knowledge of Community-Based Nurses in Supporting Parents of Preterm Babies at Home: A Survey-Based Study. *Nursing Open*, 9(3): 1883–94.

Scottish Perinatal Network Neonatal and NHS Scotland (2022) *Home Oxygen Therapy for Neonates*. [online] Available at: www.perinatalnetwork.scot/wp-content/uploads/2022/04/National-Neonatal-Network-Home-Oxygen-Guideline-V1.0.pdf (accessed 16 October 2023).

Smith, V C, Love, K and Goyer, E (2022) NICU Discharge Preparation and Transition Planning: Guidelines and Recommendations. *Journal of Perinatology*, 42(Suppl 1): 7–21.

UNICEF United Kingdom (2022) *Guide to the UNICEF UK Baby Friendly Initiative Neonatal Standards*. [online] Available at: www.unicef.org.uk/babyfriendly/wp-content/uploads/sites/2/2022/03/UNICEF-UK-Baby-Friendly-Initiative-Guide-to-the-Neonatal-Standards.pdf (accessed 17 October 2023).

14 Growth and development of the infant in neonatal care and the first year of life

Julia Petty

INTRODUCTION

While survival of very premature infants has increased in the past 20 years, the potential for significant morbidity continues, including lifelong disabilities (Petty et al, 2018; World Health Organization, 2023a) as well as developmental and behavioural problems later in life (UCL, EPICure study, 2023). Premature birth and dealing with illness and hospitalisation in the early weeks of life can affect the way infants develop in the first year of life, a critical period of brain development. In neonatal care, it is common to see infants born with restricted weight and poor growth trajectories. This chapter covers the range of terminology relating to birth weights, the issue of faltering growth and altered development expectations (Figures 14.1 to 14.3; Tables 14.1 to 14.3), as they apply to the sick and/or premature infant in the first year of life.

Chapter learning objectives

By the end of this chapter you will:

✓ have considered the importance of monitoring growth and development in infants born prematurely or who require further attention due to sickness;

✓ have a greater understanding of the developmental expectations of infants who have gone home from the neonatal unit, in the first year of life.

Critical thinking points

- Consider what factors influence the growth and development of premature infants compared to those born at term.

- Think about why healthcare professionals and parents require knowledge of the reasons for faltering growth and adjusted milestones in relation to corrected gestion.

 For growth and development relating to the healthy term infant, please refer to Chapter 3. Developmental care in the neonatal unit is covered in Chapter 9.

GROWTH

Infants born prematurely or those that have been hospitalised in the early days of life can display atypical growth and development.

Weight

Weight is regularly measured and plotted for all infants throughout the stay on the neonatal unit at a greater frequency compared to healthy infants, since weight is an important parameter that guides prescribed feed volumes and fluid management. Infants in the neonatal unit commonly lose weight and change/drop centiles if they are sick and spend significant time in hospital. Despite best efforts at prevention, weight in premature infants can show a downward centile crossing after birth (Cole et al, 2014). Similarly, centiles may increase. Nutritional management must consider these situations and be optimised appropriately. Accelerated growth should be avoided.

Birth weight is also an important parameter at birth. Low birth weight of varying degrees (Figure 14.1) can ensue due to being born early and can be influenced by maternal factors including placental function and interference with foetal growth. Normal intrauterine growth is 10–15 grams/kg/day (Sharma et al, 2016), although preterm neonates rarely achieve this. Weight should also be considered in association with gestational age (Figure 14.2). Infants who are growth restricted have similar potential problems to those born prematurely but there are also some differences – it is important to understand the latter to guide management appropriately for infants that present in the neonatal with low birth weights (Table 14.1).

Stop and think

Weight in line with gestation can be monitored during pregnancy by scanning in the second and third trimester. This may identify at-risk neonates.

Low birthweight (LBW)

- **LBW:** Low birth weight (<2.5 kg)
- **VLBW:** Very low birth weight (<1.5 kg)
- **ELBW:** Extremely low birth weight (<1 kg)

Weight and gestational age

- **AGA:** Appropriate for gestational age – growth is as expected for gestation
- **SGA:** Small for gestational age; also called 'small for dates' – growth is less than expected for gestation (< 10th centile)
- **LGA:** Large for gestational age; Growth is more than expected for gestation > 90th centile (eg Macrosomia)
- **See also Figure 14.2 for a graphical representation of weight and gestational age in relation to centiles**

Intrauterine growth restriction (IUGR)

- **IUGR:** Intra-uterine growth restriction. Growth that is not permitted to reach the maximum growth potential due to problems during pregnancy.
- **SYMMETRICAL IUGR:** Growth restriction that is proportional for both head and body: ie both are small and have remained so throughout pregnancy. Causes: genetic, chromosomal or congenital infection.
- **ASYMMETRICAL IUGR:** Growth restriction whereby head / brain growth is within expected norms but the body growth is reduced – ie head and body are disproportionate. Causes: poor placental function hindering transfer of nutrients and oxygen to the foetus.

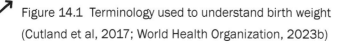

Figure 14.1 Terminology used to understand birth weight (Cutland et al, 2017; World Health Organization, 2023b)

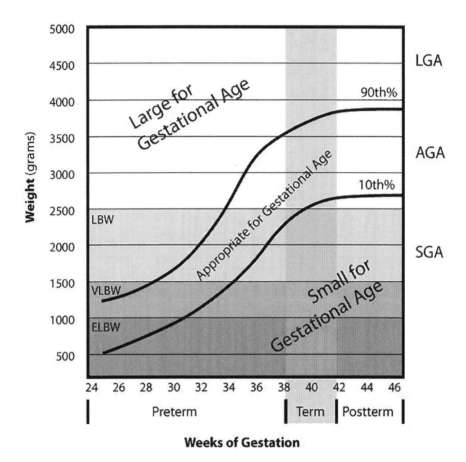

Figure 14.2 Weight and gestational age in relation to centiles

Table 14.1 Guide to distinguishing growth restricted and preterm neonates (<34 weeks)

	Differences	
Assessment feature	**Preterm**	**Intrauterine growth restriction (IUGR)**
Physiological systems	Immature.	Mature (as for term).
Airway and breathing	Surfactant deficiency and pulmonary immaturity/ insufficiency.	Lungs in alveolar stage of development and producing surfactant.

	Differences	
Assessment feature	**Preterm**	**Intrauterine growth restriction (IUGR)**
Gastro-intestinal tract	Poor suck/swallow reflex. Unable to feed orally.	Able to suck and swallow and feed normally. Often very hungry with lusty cry.
Musculoskeletal system	Poor tone and flat, extended posture.	Physiological flexion formed, good muscle tone, flexed limbs.
Pinna of ear	No cartilage and floppy.	Cartilage is formed.
Nipple	Not raised.	Raised.
Sole of foot	Smooth.	Creases evident.
Skin	Red and shiny (very preterm).	Formed skin with keratin present.
	Fragile. Lacks keratin.	May be baggy due to reduced subcutaneous fat.
	Similarities	
Weight	<2.5 kg	<2.5 kg
Thermoregulation	Poor thermal control.	Poor thermal control.
Blood glucose	Lack of glycogen reserves and at risk of hypoglycaemia.	Lack of glycogen reserves and at risk of hypoglycaemia.
Nutrition	Lack of nutritional reserves from pregnancy.	Lack of nutritional reserves from pregnancy.

 Stop and think

It is important to know if a small infant is that way due to intrauterine growth restriction, immaturity or both.

Faltering growth

For infants requiring more frequent assessment, there are specific growth charts dedicated to these specific needs designed for plotting growth measurements of premature and low birth weight infants from 23 weeks' gestation to the corrected age of two years, and for other infants requiring closer monitoring (Royal College of Paediatrics and Child Health (RCPCH), 2009, 2011, 2023; Norris et al, 2018).

Figure 14.3 is an example of a growth chart for premature infants. Table 14.2 outlines the current guidance for infants where growth is faltering (National Institute for Health and Care Excellence (NICE), 2017).

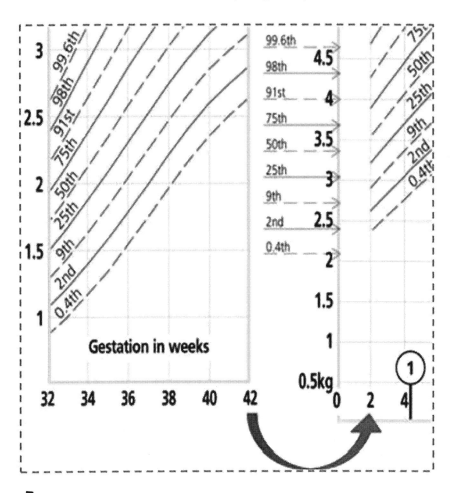

↗ Figure 14.3 Preterm growth chart

© Royal College of Paediatrics and Child Health

☙ Stop and think

It is important to plot weight in very premature infants (born less than 36 weeks and 6 days only) using **gestational correction** that adjusts the plot for the number of weeks a baby was born early.

- Number of weeks early = 40 weeks minus gestational age at birth. This is continued until one year for infants born at 32–36 weeks and two years for infants born before 32 weeks. Infants over 36 weeks and 6 days are considered 'term' so gestational correction should not be used.

 Table 14.2 Current guidance for infants where growth is faltering

Be aware that the following factors may be associated with faltering growth:
- preterm birth;
- neurodevelopmental concerns;
- maternal postnatal depression or anxiety.

Recognise that in faltering growth, a range of factors may contribute to the problem, and it may not be possible to identify a clear cause. There may be difficulties in the interaction between an infant or child and the parents or carers that may contribute to the problem.

Based on the feeding history, consider the following:
- ineffective suckling in breastfed infants;
- ineffective bottle feeding;
- feeding environment and possible aversion;
- parent/carer–infant interactions;
- how parents respond to the infant's feeding cues;
- physical disorders that affect feeding.

Consider using the following as thresholds for concern about faltering growth in infants and children (a centile space being the space between adjacent centile lines on the UK WHO growth charts):
- a fall across weight centiles;
- when current weight is below the second centile for age, whatever the birth weight.

Interventions
- Measurement of weight and height or length.
- Plot the above measurements and available previous measurements on the UK WHO growth charts to assess weight change and linear growth over time.
- Feeding support.
- Consider nutrient fortification.
- Close monitoring.
- Referral.
- Consider enteral tube feeding only when other interventions have been tried without improvement.

For full guidance on interventions refer to the NICE guidance (2017).

(NICE, 2017)

ASSESSING GROWTH AND DEVELOPMENTAL MILESTONES IN THE PREMATURE INFANT

Reaching developmental milestones may take longer for premature infants by comparison with babies born at full term. This is because they are younger. When assessing the development of a child who has been born prematurely, it is therefore necessary to review them against the expected milestones for their *corrected* age (Table 14.3) – this is worked out by calculating their age from their *original* due date, rather than the date they were born. Correction is not necessary once the child reaches the age of two years (Lissaur and Claydon, 2018).

 Table 14.3 Adjusted developmental milestones in premature infants in the first year of life

At birth
There may be weak or absent reflexes, depending on gestation, eg immature suck/swallow co-ordination. In very premature infants, movement may be limited or immature due to lack of muscle tone and eyes may be fused.

At 1 month corrected
Infants may wave their arms and legs when they are on their back, turn their head when they are on their tummy, watch their hands as they move them. They may cry when they are hungry and make cooing sounds.

At 4 months corrected
They may move their head from side to side when they are on their back, hold their head up and hold their head steady, stop crying when they hear a voice, smile or coo, make sounds when looking at toys or people.

At 6 months corrected
They lift their legs high enough to see their feet when they are on their back, support their own weight while standing if you are holding their hands, make sounds and react differently towards strangers than they do with familiar people.

At 7 months corrected
They get into the crawling position by getting on their hands and knees, sit up straight for several minutes without using their hands and support, hold on to furniture without leaning their chest against it for support, babble, respond to the tone of voice and stop what they are doing.

At 9 months corrected
They can walk beside furniture while holding on with only one hand, pick up a small toy with only one hand, put a small toy down without dropping it, say three words, such as 'mama', 'dada' and 'baba', and follow simple commands such as 'come here', 'give it to me' or 'put it back'.

At 12 months corrected
They may take several steps without tripping or falling while standing (if you are holding both hands), help turn pages of a book, look at an object when you ask them where it is, play with a doll or cuddly toy by hugging it, and roll or throw a toy at you so you can return it.

For full parental guidance, see Tommy's (2021).

Stop and think

As highlighted in Chapter 3, always consider individual differences and advise parents of this, especially if they compare their infant with another. Parents can be advised to use milestones positively in different ways: eg if their infant starts to roll over from about two months, they can give them a helping hand.

 See the web companion for a glossary specific to this chapter.

 Check local variations and guidance alert

The space below can be used to record any notes or local variations and practice points specific to your own unit.

REFERENCES

Cole, T J, Statnikov, Y, Santhakumaran, S, Pan, H and Modi, N (2014) Neonatal Data Analysis Unit and the Preterm Growth Investigator Group. Birth Weight and Longitudinal Growth in Infants Born below 32 Weeks' Gestation: A UK Population Study. *Archives of Disease in Childhood. Fetal and Neonatal Edition*, 99(1): F34–F40.

Cutland, C L, Lackritz, E M, Mallett-Moore, T et al, and the Brighton Collaboration Low Birth Weight Working Group (2017) Low Birth Weight: Case Definition & Guidelines for Data Collection, Analysis, and Presentation of Maternal Immunization Safety Data. *Vaccine*, 35(48): 6492–500.

Lissauer, T and Claydon, W (2018) *Illustrated Textbook of Paediatrics*. 5th ed. Oxford: Elsevier.

National Institute for Health and Care Excellence (NICE) (2017) Faltering Growth: Recognition and Management of Faltering Growth in Children. NICE Guideline [NG75]. [online] Available at: www.nice.org.uk/guidance/ng75 (accessed 1 November 2023).

Norris, T, Seaton, S E, Manktelow, B N et al (2018) Updated Birth Weight Centiles for England and Wales. *Archives of Disease in Childhood. Fetal and Neonatal Edition*, 103: F577–F582.

Petty, J, Whiting, L, Green, J and Fowler, C (2018) Parents' Views on Preparation to Care for Premature Infants at Home. *Nursing Children & Young People*, 30(4): 22–7.

Royal College of Paediatrics and Child Health (RCPCH) (2009) *Plotting Preterm Infants: Fact Sheet 5*. [online] Available at: www.rcpch.ac.uk/sites/default/files/Plotting_preterm_infants.pdf (accessed 1 November 2023).

Royal College of Paediatrics and Child Health (RCPCH) (2011) *Neonatal and Infant Close Monitoring Growth Chart (NICM): Fact Sheet 7*. [online] Available at: www.rcpch.ac.uk/sites/default/files/Plotting_neonatal_and_infant_close_monitoring.pdf (accessed 1 November 2023).

Royal College of Paediatrics and Child Health (RCPCH) (2023) UK-WHO Growth Charts – Guidance for Health Professionals. [online] Available at: www.rcpch.ac.uk/resources/uk-who-growth-charts-guidance-health-professionals (accessed 1 November 2023).

Sharma, D, Shastri, S and Sharma, P (2016) Intrauterine Growth Restriction: Antenatal and Postnatal Aspects. *Clinical Medicine Insights: Pediatrics*, 10: 67–83.

Tommy's (2021) Growth and Development after Prematurity. [online] Available at: www.tommys.org/pregnancy-information/premature-birth/taking-your-baby-home/growth-and-development-after-prematurity (accessed 1 November 2023).

University College London (UCL), EPICure study (2023) About – Premature Babies: A Success Story. [online] Available at: www.ucl.ac.uk/womens-health/research/neonatology/epicure/about (accessed 1 November 2023).

World Health Organization (WHO) (2023a) Preterm Birth. [online] Available at: www.who.int/news-room/fact-sheets/detail/preterm-birth (accessed 1 November 2023).

World Health Organization (WHO) (2023b) Low Birth Weight. [online] Available at: www.who.int/data/nutrition/nlis/info/low-birth-weight (accessed 1 November 2023).

Community-based family care

Karen Roberts-Edema (Queen's Nurse)

INTRODUCTION

The role of the neonatal community team, often known as outreach, is to provide support to infants with complex healthcare needs. Community-based neonatal care using careful discharge planning aims not only to reduce the length of stay in hospital for the infant and their parents, but also to continue tailored support at home. There is an increased survival rate for premature infants born before 37 weeks' completed gestation. Premature infants may experience an array of health conditions relating to their immaturity of vital organs, often requiring additional support from community teams. These preterm infants ultimately require assistance once they have been discharged from hospital (Spence et al, 2023). To reduce the length of stay or readmissions, the community neonatal nurse (CNN) supports the infant and family to transition home. Depending on the area in which the family is living in, the CNN will support the infant and family from a range of a few days up to six weeks and in some areas up to six months. Once this period has elapsed then the infant will be transferred to the Children's Community Nursing Team (Boykova and Kenner, 2012).

The role of the community children's nurse (CCN) is flexible, diverse, dynamic, and responsive to children and young people and their families. The CCN will support children and young people in the home and in the school setting. The CCN's philosophy is to provide care to children and young people and empower families to care for their children in the home. This includes acute, short-term, complex, technology-dependent long-term conditions, as well as children and young people with disabilities, complex conditions which may require continuing healthcare, and neonates (The Queen's Nursing Institute, 2018). This chapter covers discharge planning, assessment in the home, supporting parents at home, the role of community and/or outreach services and a consideration of ongoing risk and safeguarding (Figures 15.1 to 15.2; Tables 15.1 to 15.6).

Chapter learning objectives

By the end of this chapter you will:

✓ understand the role of the community neonatal nurse and children's community nurse in caring for the family after discharge home;

✓ understand the assessment required when a child is at home;

✓ understand the support the parents need to care for infants in the community.

Critical thinking points

• Consider the assessment of the parents and their needs and what support they would require to ensure their child does not get readmitted to hospital.

• What equipment is essential for a safe transition home?

 See Chapter 13 for further information on discharge planning and transition of the infant from neonatal care to home.

 See the web companion for supplementary information relating to parental support in the community.

DISCHARGE PLANNING

Discharge planning is an essential part of the infant's journey; each neonatal unit has a unique approach to arranging discharge planning for families. The discharge planning includes the availability of resources within the local area and specific basic information, which will help the smooth transition from hospital to home (Smith et al, 2022). The essential information will help the CNN and CCN team to ensure the holistic care of the infant at home (Purdy et al, 2015). Some infants will be technology dependent; therefore, a robust discharge plan needs to be in place to care for those children (Whiting, 2019). Table 15.1 and Figure 15.1 are a checklist and a flow chart, respectively, of what to expect when an infant is being discharged home. Table 15.2 covers assessment in the home environment.

Table 15.1 Checklist for transition to home

This checklist needs to be considered before the infant transitions home.

- Co-ordinated care from a specialist healthcare provider CNN or CCN.

- Discharge summary to include medication summary.

- Weaning oxygen regime – if infant is on home oxygen.

- Feeding regime.

- Feeding difficulties: nasogastric tube size, date of insertion.

- Follow-up appointments pending.

- Ongoing monitoring of immunisations.

- Developmental screening.

- High-risk infants to have access to specialist professionals.

- Equipment list and requirements.

- If developmental delay is suspected, follow up with paediatrician.

- Behaviour of the infant – advise on strategies to cope with an infant at home.

- Identify training and development needs for parents.

Discharge from hospital. Referral to Community Neonatal or Children's Community Nursing team.

Visit/contact from CNN/CCN within 24 to 48 hours (depending on the local area).

Initial visit. Full assesment by both medical and social services.

Equipment preparation. Map out the timeline for transition to other services.

Communicate the emergency contact details to parents:
Co-ordination of care/name of nurse
Advice/follow-up visit

Figure 15.1 Flow chart for discharge home
(Department of Health, 2011)

⊞ Table 15.2 Neonatal assessment at home

Referral from	
Patient details	**Home environment**
Name	Flat
DOB	House
Parent name(s)	Who lives in the home
Mother	Smokers in the home
Father	Pets
Language spoken at home	Smoke and carbon monoxide alarms
	Home oxygen arrangements

Infant assessment	
Nutrition	**Physical assessment**
Oral feeds	Fontanelle
Breastfeeding	Skin
NGT feeds	Mouth
Size of tube	Eyes
Type of tube	Abdomen
When tube was inserted	Vital signs – ▐➤ see Chapters 4 and 10
Education on tube changing and feeding	

Equipment requirements

Equipment list

Consumables

Referrals as/if required, to

✓ Social services

✓ Speech and language therapy

✓ Physiotherapy

✓ Occupational therapy

✓ Health visitor

✓ Mental health services

✓ Safeguarding concerns, if required

Adapted from Division of Public Health Women's and Children Health Section (2010)

SUPPORT FOR PARENTS AT HOME

Community support is essential for parents after they have transitioned home (Petty et al, 2018, 2019, 2022). It is important to remember that the neonatal outreach service is different from one area to the next in the United Kingdom. The neonatal journey maybe a complex one whereby the infant will encounter several services; parents therefore need support in navigating these services. Tables 15.3 to 15.5 outline key points in relation to supporting parents.

 Table 15.3 Role of the outreach team

Some areas have a neonatal outreach programme. This is where the neonatal team see the infants at home after discharge to help reduce readmission into hospital. The outreach team supports parents with several complexities, such as arranging home oxygen and managing feeding whether that is breastfeeding, oral feeding or enteral feeding. They train the parents to give medication and monitor their infant's progress, give advice on ongoing medical needs and ensure the parents are aware of how to obtain help if needed.

(Smith et al, 2022)

> **Check local guidance**
>
> Not all areas have a neonatal outreach team; information on what an area provides can be found on the NHS website where the neonatal unit is situated.

⊞ Table 15.4 Support for parents at home

Support in the community

Who to contact for support:

- CNN or CCN;
- specialist nurse;
- GP;
- social services for financial, housing support.

When to contact support networks:

- local CNN and CCN times may vary according to area;
- CNN/CCN team may have an on-call service;
- local hospital ward 24-hour access – sometimes called open access depending on the area;
- GP – local GP hours.

Why contact professionals:

- expert advice for medical reasons;
- GP for advice, referrals and repeat medications;
- decision making and reassurance;
- troubleshooting equipment or medical condition.

How to contact support networks:

- CNN/CCN office number;
- 999/112;
- CNN/CCN mobile phone number;
- video calls/clinics/Hospital @ Home.

(Adapted from Whiting, 2019)

The use of technology in the community

- The NHS Long Term Plan (2019) set out a vision to have person-centred services, which will include virtual wards and hospital at home services to support patients at home.
- Once the infant is transferred to the CCN team, the parents and family may experience a hospital at home service.
- The hospital at home service can be delivered via telephone, online consultations (with the use of iPads and laptops), clinic-based care or home visits (Royal College of Nursing (RCN), 2020).
- This is to reduce readmissions to hospital and to provide improved service and patient care.

Charities and hospice care

Bliss charity provides:

- emotional and practical support;
- information about parents' mental health;
- financial information;
- support for LGBTQIA+ families;
- help with coping with loss and bereavement;
- palliative care;
- help with making critical decisions.

Lullaby charity provides:

- sleep advice for infants;
- advice on multiple births;
- a chance to share the neonatal experience of having a premature infant;
- training and advice;
- bereavement services.

→

Table 15.4 (cont.)

Together for Short Lives provides:

- help for parents to understand the diagnosis;
- ongoing care and support;
- family resources;
- families with the ability to connect with other families with similar experiences;
- end-of-life care;
- bereavement services.

Hospices provide:

- 24-hour telephone support;
- practice help, advice and information;
- specialist short break care;
- specialist therapies: – physiotherapy, complementary therapies and play and music therapy;
- 24-hour end-of-life care;
- care for a child after death;
- training for parents.

 Stop and think

Consider the family as a whole unit. Families are made up of different religions, backgrounds, races and cultures. Think what is appropriate for each individual family.

 Table 15.5 Summary of support for parents

There are many services to support parents to care for their infant within the community. It is important that the infants and their families are referred to the correct service or signposted to the support networks that will help the transition from hospital to home go smoothly. Many of these families have been on the neonatal unit for some time and therefore they are used to 24-hour care; it can be daunting for a family to be discharged home and feel they do not have the correct support to help them. If a child has ongoing complex needs, there are charities and a children's hospice to help them. A children's hospice is there to support families when their child is at the end of their lives. However, some hospices provide short break services and community services to care for the child with complex needs at home.

Stop and think

Signposting parents to support services such as charities and/or peer support networks is vital. Community teams should signpost families to the appropriate resource, service and/or organisation after their needs are assessed. See Chapter 16.

IDENTIFYING RISK AT HOME

To ensure safety at home and provide reassurance for parents relating to caring for their infant, identifying areas of risk is essential. A lack of consistency in care and communication across community teams can result in increased parental stress. This adds to the stress caused by the specific vulnerability of their infant relating to, for example, an increased risk of being re-hospitalised and a higher chance of infection, along with the risks associated with complex needs, tube feeding and home oxygen. Figure 15.2 and Table 15.6 provide a brief overview of considerations relating to risk.

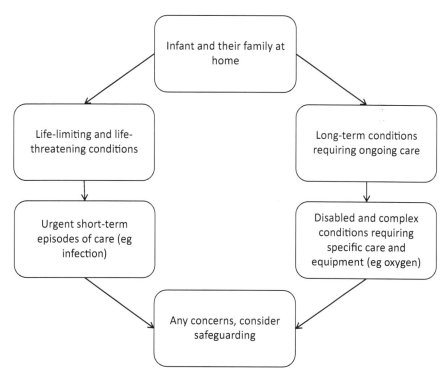

Figure 15.2 Risks in the home

(HM Government, 2018)

Stop and think

Children with complex health needs and disabilities are vulnerable to abuse. Social care provides support to vulnerable children and their families. A social care referral should be made to see if there is support the infant and family can receive while at home.

 Table 15.6 Summary of safeguarding

The welfare of children is paramount, and it is the practitioner's duty to ensure their patients do not suffer any significant harm. All professionals who encounter children and their families have a duty of care to safeguard children. Therefore, consider how to protect children from maltreatment, preventing impairment of their mental and physical development. Ensuring children grow up in a safe environment and enabling them to grow to their full potential is the duty of all professionals who encounter them.

It is imperative that professionals are aware of their role when caring for an infant/child in the community and understand how to escalate concerns if they arise (HM Government, 2018).

 ### Standard precautions alert

Parents also need education and advice on infection prevention as their infant may be more susceptible due to being premature or having complex needs – for example, good hygiene, handwashing and observing for worrying signs along with how and who to report these to.

 See Chapter 16 for useful parent and health professional resources.

 See the web companion for supplementary information throughout this chapter and for a glossary specific to this chapter.

Check local variations and guidance alert

The space below can be used to record any notes, local variations and practice points specific to your own unit.

REFERENCES

Bliss (nd) Medical Support When You Go Home. [online] Available at: www.bliss.org.uk/parents/going-home-from-the-neonatal-unit/medical-support-when-you-go-home-from-the-neonatal-unit (accessed 5 December 2023).

Boykova, M and Kenner, C (2012) Transition from Hospital to Home for Parents of Preterm Infants. *The Journal of Perinatal and Neonatal Nursing*, 26(1): 81–7.

Department of Health (2011) *NHS at Home: Community Children's Nursing Services*. [online] Available at: https://assets.publishing.service.gov.uk/media/5a74aa2ee5274a52940692e1/dh_124900.pdf (accessed 5 December 2023).

Division of Public Health Women's and Children Health Section (2010) Protocol: Home Visit for Newborn Care and Assessment. London: DHHS.

HM Government (2018) *Working Together to Safeguard Children: A Guide to Inter-agency Working to Safeguard and Promote the Welfare of Children*. London: HM Government.

Lullaby Trust (nd) Safer Sleep for Babies, Support for Families. [online] Available at: www.lullabytrust.org.uk (accessed 5 December 2023).

National Health Service (NHS) (2019) NHS Long Term Plan. [online] Available at: www.longtermplan.nhs.uk (accessed 28 January 2024).

Petty, J, Whiting, L, Green, J and Fowler, C (2018) Parents' Views on Preparation to Care for Extremely Premature Infants at Home. *Nursing Children and Young People*, 30(4): 22–7.

Petty, J, Whiting, L, Mosenthal, A, Fowler, C, Elliott, D and Green, J (2019) The Knowledge and Learning Needs of Health Professionals in Providing Support for Parents of Premature Babies at Home: A Mixed-Methods Study. *Journal of Neonatal Nursing*, 25(6): 277–84.

Petty, J, Whiting, L, Green, J and Fowler, C (2022) Exploring the Knowledge of Community-Based Nurses in Supporting Parents of Preterm Babies at Home: A Survey-Based Study. *Nursing Open*, 9(3): 1883–94.

Queen's Nursing Institute (2018) *The QNI/QNIS Voluntary Standards for Community Children's Nurse Education Practice*. London: The Queen's Nursing Institute.

Royal College of Nursing (2020) *Futureproofing Community Children's Nursing*. London: RCN.

Smith, V C, Love, K and Goyer, E (2022) NICU Discharge Preparation Planning: Guidelines and Recommendations. *Journal of Perinatology*, 42: 7–21.

Spence, C M, Stuyvenberg, C L, Kane, A E, Burnsed J and Dusing, S C (2023) Parent Experiences in the NICU and Transition to Home. *International Journal of Environmental Research and Public Health*, 20(11). https://doi.org/10.3390/ijerph20116050.

Together for Short Lives (TFSL) (2022) What Is Children's Palliative Care and Hospice Care? [online] Available at: www.togetherforshortlives.org.uk/what-is-childrens-palliative-and-hospice-care (accessed 5 December 2023).

Whiting, M (2019) Caring for Children – '24-7': The Experience of WellChild Nurses and the Families for whom They Are Providing Care and Support. *Journal of Child Health Care*, 23(1): 35–44.

16 Resources for health professionals and parents

Karen Afford and Julia Petty

INTRODUCTION

This book has emphasised that for infants requiring specialist care, parents and families play a crucial role in supporting their well-being. To ensure the best outcomes for these vulnerable infants, it is essential for health professionals and parents to have access to reliable and comprehensive resources that guide their knowledge and understanding of neonatal care and the unique needs of infants and families. This chapter presents a selected, curated list of resources that cover various aspects of neonatal care, offering evidence-based knowledge to support healthcare professionals and parents alike.

Chapter learning objectives

By the end of this chapter you will:

- ✓ have gained a collection of resources for your own further reading and for you to refer parents and learners to;

- ✓ be able to signpost parents and learners within the neonatal team to a range of useful resources to support practice.

Critical thinking points

- Consider any other resources to add to those within this chapter.

- What are the most useful and informative resources for your own evidence-based knowledge enhancement and how would you signpost these to others?

 Refer to all chapters for their specific supporting literature.

See the web companion for further reading and resources on all aspects of neonatal care.

SOURCES OF INFORMATION

Peer-reviewed journals and articles

Journals and research articles serve as authoritative sources of information for health professionals seeking evidence-based knowledge. The following are suggested publications that feature articles on neonatal health, covering topics such as neonatal intensive care, feeding, neurodevelopment and family-centred care. These resources provide valuable insights into cutting-edge research and best practices. Selected examples include:

o   *Journal of Neonatal Nursing:* www.sciencedirect.com/journal/journal-of-neonatal-nursing

o   *Journal of Health Visiting:* www.magsubscriptions.com/healthcare-nursing-journal-of-health-visiting-journal-of-health-visiting-print-website-cpd

o   *Archives of Disease in Childhood (Fetal and Neonatal Edition):* https://fn.bmj.com

o   *Advances in Neonatal Care:* https://journals.lww.com/advancesinneonatalcare/pages/default.aspx

o   *Journal of Obstetric, Gynecologic & Neonatal Nursing:* www.jognn.org

o   *Infant journal:* www.infantjournal.co.uk/default.html

o   *Birth journal:* https://onlinelibrary.wiley.com/journal/1523536x

o   *Journal of Perinatal and Neonatal Nursing:* https://journals.lww.com/jpnnjournal/pages/default.aspx

o   *Nursing Children & Young People:* https://journals.rcni.com/nursing-children-and-young-people

Professional associations and guidelines

The national or global organisations below are reputable sources of knowledge relating to child and neonatal health.

o   Neonatal Nurses Association (UK), representing the voice of neonatal nurses across the UK: www.nna.org.uk

○ The Institute of Health Visiting (iHV) offers a wealth of invaluable information and support to new parents, aiming to promote the health and well-being of families during the crucial early years of a child's life. Their services encompass various aspects of parenting: https://ihv.org.uk

○ The British Association of Perinatal Medicine (BAPM): an organisation representing professionals that work in perinatal care, including neonatal and obstetric doctors, nurses, advanced neonatal nurse practitioners (ANNPs), midwives, managers and allied health professionals: www.bapm.org

○ Royal Society of Paediatrics and Child Health (RCPCH): www.rcpch. ac.uk/resources

○ National Institute for Health and Care Excellence (NICE): publishes guidelines and recommendations for neonatal care. These guidelines offer health professionals and parents a standardised approach to managing various neonatal conditions, promoting uniformity and improved outcomes: www.nice.org.uk

○ The Council of International Neonatal Nurses (COINN): www.coinnurses. org/resources

○ Community of Neonatal Nursing Practice (CoNP): www. conpcommunityofpractice.org/resources

○ European Standards of Care for Newborn Health: www.efcni.org/ activities/projects/escnh

○ European Foundation for the Care of Newborn Infants (EFCNI): www. efcni.org/activities/projects

○ Global Alliance of Newborn Health: www.efcni.org/activities/projects/ glance-global-alliance-for-newborn-care

○ The World Health Organization: www.who.int/news-room/fact-sheets/ detail/preterm-birth

○ UNICEF: www.unicef.org.uk/babyfriendly/baby-friendly-resources

Neonatal care books

Books dedicated to neonatal care are valuable resources for health professionals and parents seeking in-depth knowledge. Below is a list of recent neonatal textbooks (published within the past five years).

○ Boxwell, G, Petty, J and Kaiser, L (eds) (2020) *Neonatal Intensive Care Nursing*. 3rd ed. Routledge.

o   Davies, L and McDonald, S (2020) *Examination of the Newborn and Neonatal Health.* 2nd ed. Elsevier.

o   Edwards, A (2020) *Postnatal & Neonatal Midwifery Skills: Survival Guide.* 2nd ed. Routledge.

o   Gardner, S L and Carter, B S (2020) *Merenstein & Gardner's Handbook of Neonatal Intensive Care: An Interprofessional Approach.* 9th ed. Elsevier.

o   Jones, T (2019) *The Student Guide to the Newborn Infant Physical Examination.* Routledge.

o   Kain, V (ed) and Mannix, T (2022) *Neonatal Care for Nurses and Midwives: Principles for Practice.* 2nd ed. Elsevier.

o   Kenner, C and Boykova, M V (2021) *Neonatal Nursing Care Handbook: An Evidence-Based Approach to Conditions and Procedures.* 3rd ed. Springer.

o   Petty, J, Jones, T, van den Hoogen, A, Walker, K and Kenner, C (eds) (2022) *Neonatal Nursing: A Global Perspective.* Springer.

Online courses and webinars

Various platforms offer online courses and webinars for health professionals to enhance their understanding of neonatal care. The Neonatal Nurses Association (NNA UK) and BAPM deliver regular webinars on a range of topics for their members (membership fee applies with member benefits). Free neonatal courses are offered through NHS England's E-learning for Health platform (free to register providing that you have an NHS or a university email address) – https://portal.e-lfh.org.uk. Topics covered include Atain ('Avoiding Term Admissions to Neonatal Care'), neonatal jaundice, blood glucose monitoring, thermoregulation and bonding/attachment. FutureLearn runs an online course on newborn assessment – www.futurelearn.com/courses/neonatal-assessment.

Courses are also offered on the following areas.

o   Creating nurturing sensory environments for infants and families by Sensory Beginnings: https://sensorybeginnings.com/why-sensory

o   Family and Infant Neurodevelopmental Education (FINE): www.finetraininguk.com

o   Neonatal Individualised Developmental Care Assessment programme (NIDCAP): https://nidcap.org/trainingcenter/uk-nidcap-training-center

Parenting websites, social media platforms and support groups

Additionally, joining support groups like the NICU Parent Network and online forums allows parents to connect with others who have similar experiences, fostering a sense of community and emotional support. The UK Operational Delivery Networks (ODNs) offer a variety of resources and support to both parents and health professionals. BAPM provides a list of all ODNs here: www. bapm.org/pages/19-neonatal-networks.

There are also a range of parent support charities:

- Bliss: www.bliss.org.uk
- Tiny Life: www.tinylife.org.uk
- Leo's: https://leosneonatal.org
- Spoons: https://spoons.org.uk/
- Noah's Star: https://noahsstar.co.uk
- Born Too Soon: https://borntoosoon.org.uk/family-friends-support-for-neonatal-charity
- Stillbirth and Neonatal Death Society (Sands): www.sands.org.uk
- Lullaby Trust: www.lullabytrust.org.uk
- FICare™: https://familyintegratedcare.com

Neonatal health apps

Several mobile applications offer quick references and tools for neonatal care. Apps like NIPE, NeoMate, Neonatal Resuscitation, Growth Charts UK-WHO, Tommy's charity, 'Healthier Together' and 'Ages and Stages' provide healthcare professionals and/or parents with dosing calculators, growth charts and clinical guidelines at their fingertips.

- www.cambridgedigitalhealth.co.uk/nipe-app
- https://qicentral.rcpch.ac.uk/medsiq/safe-prescribing/neomate
- www.resus.org.uk/library/iresus
- https://growthchart.app
- www.tommys.org/pregnancy-information/premature-birth/my-prem-baby-app
- www.what0-18.nhs.uk/parentscarers/worried-your-child-unwell
- https://agesandstages.com/landing-page/calculator-app

Educational videos and infographics

Visual resources, such as educational videos and infographics, can be valuable tools for both health professionals and parents delivered through platforms like YouTube and Patient Story sites.

o   'Stories from the Neonatal Unit' – parent-focused digital stories: https://neonatalstories.com. Click on the parent stories tab.

o   The 'Patient Voices' neonatal page – Parent Voices digital stories: www.patientvoices.org.uk/naoneo.htm

o   NICU Foundation – 'A Stay in Neonatal Care': https://youtu.be/ARYFMnXhmLw?si=B7Y43zNLHHhFuh_v

o   University of Hertfordshire – 'Appreciation of the Neonatal Unit Through the Eyes/Stories of Student Nurses': www.health.herts.ac.uk/elearning/petty/neonate/nav

USEFUL WEBSITES

The table below has some specific web-based resources listed, useful for either parents, health professionals or both. It is not an exhaustive list so do add your own in the space provided at the end.

Website	Subject	Link
Neonatal Intensive Care Nursing book student web-based companion site	A variety of neonatal care topics for anyone working in the field	https://routledgetextbooks.com/textbooks/9781138556843
The Institute for Health Visiting (iHV)	Transition to parenthood	https://ihv.org.uk/for-health-visitors/resources-for-members/resource/ihv-tips-for-parents/transition-to-parenthood-and-the-early-weeks/pt-accessing-health-visiting-support-for-you-and-your-family
iHV	Managing minor illness	https://ihv.org.uk/for-health-visitors/resources-for-members/resource/ihv-tips-for-parents/managing-minor-illness-and-reducing-accidents/oral-thrush
NHS childhood vaccinations	Additional reading: the following web pages give further helpful advice on childhood vaccinations.	www.nhs.uk/conditions/vaccinations

Website	Subject	Link
UK guidance on immunisations	Leaflets and guidance on immunisations for parents of premature babies.	www.gov.uk/government/publications/a-quick-guide-to-childhood-immunisation-for-the-parents-of-premature-babies
Healthier Together	Unwell child over three months.	www.what0-18.nhs.uk/parentscarers/worried-your-child-unwell
Jaundice awareness	Guidance for parents and professionals on managing and monitoring jaundice.	https://childliverdisease.org/yellow-alert
Birth to 5 Matters	*Birth to 5 Matters* has been developed by the Early Years Coalition, composed of the 16 early years sector organisations.	https://birthto5matters.org.uk
Gov.org	Early years.	www.gov.uk/early-years-foundation-stage
Early Years Alliance	Early years.	www.eyalliance.org.uk/early-years-foundation-stage
Parent helplines		www.youngminds.org.uk/parent/parents-helpline-and-webchat
Bliss (UK baby charity)	This charity offers vital support to parents of premature babies –emotional guidance, resources and information to help parents navigate their sometimes-challenging journey.	www.bliss.org.uk/parents/support
Tommy's charity UK	Developmental milestones according to 'corrected age'.	www.tommys.org/pregnancy-information/premature-birth/taking-your-baby-home/growth-and-development-after-prematurity
The Children's Trust charity	A free online resource has launched to help school staff and educational professionals support children who were born before 37 weeks' gestation.	www.thechildrenstrust.org.uk/brain-injury-information/latest/new-learning-resource-to-help-schools-support-children-born-preterm

→

Website	Subject	Link
National Health Service (NHS) Race and Health Observatory (2023)	A review of neonatal assessment and practice in Black, Asian and minority ethnic newborns – exploring the Apgar score, the detection of cyanosis and jaundice	www.nhsrho.org/research/ review-of-neonatal-assessment- and-practice-in-black-asian-and- minority-ethnic-newborns-exploring- the-apgar-score-the-detection-of- cyanosis-and-jaundice

ADD YOUR OWN

Final words

This book is intended to support bedside nursing care of the neonate in the clinical setting. Clinical care is of course forever changing, and we should be mindful of this as we care for our vulnerable neonatal population and their families. It is imperative that we keep up to date with changes and developments in clinical practice. Some areas are continually evolving and debates have been present in relation to certain areas of practice, for example, the timing of cord clamping at birth, operational thresholds to give blood transfusions and advances in ventilation support to name just a few. In addition, supporting the emotional and communication needs of families is also a key area of ongoing interest in line with 'trauma-informed care', given how the neonatal care journey is known to be a significant source of trauma and psychological stress. Another example of vital evidence-based practice development relates to neonatal assessments, including the Apgar score, that are reported as not fit for purpose with regard to ethnic minority neonates, as discussed earlier in the book. The Preface referred to key reports that will now guide future research (EMBRACE-UK, 2023; NHSRHO, 2023), given the bias inherent in neonatal checks that can lead to inaccurate assessments, late diagnosis, and poorer outcomes in non-white neonates. This is urgent work; for example, there is a need for an immediate update of guidelines that refer to assessments by skin colour and for greater use of screening tool devices, including oximeters and bilirubinometers. Better education and training for healthcare professionals on clinical assessment of neonates from minority ethnic backgrounds is also needed. These are just examples of emerging areas of ongoing work and future research; there are of course many others which cannot be mentioned here in full.

The aim is that this book will evolve as practices change in the future. We, as editors, also hope that essential information in this book, along with the accompanying web companion, is thorough and that nothing has been missed. This includes recognition and inclusion of neonates and families from all backgrounds, races, ethnicities, cultures, gender identifies, sexual orientations, and disabilities, in line with the Equality Act (2010). We are open to suggestions in terms of the supplementary web companion content, to support the book.

REFERENCES

EMBRACE-UK (2023) MBRRACE-UK Perinatal Confidential Enquiry: A Comparison of the Care of Asian, Black and White Women Who Have Experienced a Stillbirth or Neonatal Death. [online] Available at: www.npeu.ox.ac.uk/mbrrace-uk/reports#mbrrace-uk-perinatal-confidential-enquiry-a-comparison-of-the-care-of-asian-black-and-white-women-who-have-experienced-a-stillbirth-or-neonatal-death (accessed 28 January 2024).

Equality Act 2010. [online] Available at: www.legislation.gov.uk/ukpga/2010/15/contents (accessed 5 December 2023).

National Health Service Race and Health Observatory (NHSRHO) (2023) Review of Neonatal Assessment and Practice in Black, Asian and Minority Ethnic Newborns: Exploring the Apgar Score, the Detection of Cyanosis and Jaundice. [online] Available at: www.nhsrho.org/research/review-of-neonatal-assessment-and-practice-in-black-asian-and-minority-ethnic-newborns-exploring-the-apgar-score-the-detection-of-cyanosis-and-jaundice/ (accessed 28 January 2024).

Index

Page numbers in **bold** and *italics* denote tables and figures, respectively.